1996

Mercer Guide to Social Security and Medicare

Authors

Dale R. Detlefs, B.A., B.S.C., M.B.A., J.D.
Attorney-at-Law
Former Manager, Social Security Division
William M. Mercer, Incorporated

Robert J. Myers, B.S., M.S., LL.D., F.S.A.
Consulting Actuary
Former Chief Actuary and Deputy Commissioner,
Social Security Administration

J. Robert Treanor, B.A., CEBS
Manager, Social Security Division
William M. Mercer, Incorporated

Acknowledgment

For assistance in the preparation of this book, grateful acknowledgment is made to Donna A. Clements and Suzanne Barbour.

This book is revised annually.

Are You Missing Out?

Social Security and Medicare will pay $550 billion in benefits in 1996, most of it tax free. If you aren't one of the 43 million persons getting benefits each month, you probably **are** one of the 143 million working under Social Security who can expect to receive benefits later.

If you think Social Security is just for retirement, look again. Less than half of that $550 billion for Social Security and Medicare will be paid in monthly benefits to retired workers. The rest will be paid to disabled workers; to the families of workers who have retired, become disabled, or died; and for medical expenses.

You and your employer are paying for most of those benefits right now. The self-employed pay both halves of the tax. Many families pay more Social Security and Medicare payroll taxes than federal income taxes.

Social Security taxes have increased, but so have benefits. The maximum retirement benefit at age 65 has more than doubled since 1980.

Social Security is the most important financial protection plan in the country. Any time that your income is affected by a significant event — retirement, severe disability, or death — Social Security could pay substantial benefits, which increase with the cost of living.

We've written this book to tell you in simple, practical terms what you need to know about Social Security and Medicare:

- what they **cost** you and your employer,

- what **types of benefits** they provide,

- **how much** you get,

- **when** you get it, and

- how to **make sure** you get it.

Social Security. You're paying for it today. It could be your main source of income tomorrow, if you know what to do and when to do it. Don't miss out. Read this book.

You can't afford **not** to!

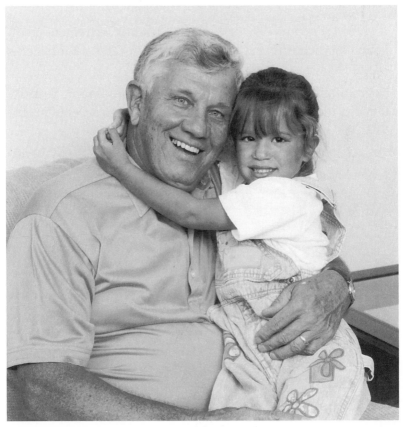

Recent Changes

New rules for 1996 result from automatic changes that occur annually and those based on past legislation. Only significant changes that might affect you or your family are explained here. Most are discussed in more detail in the text of this book on the pages indicated.

- The maximum earnings on which you pay Social Security taxes increases from $61,200 to $62,700. There is no limit on the earnings upon which you pay the Medicare tax (pages 14 and 16).

- The cost-of-living increase in benefits for December 1995, payable on January 3, 1996, is 2.6% (page 152).

- The earnings limitation for beneficiaries under age 65 increases from $8,160 to $8,280; for beneficiaries at ages 65-69, it increases from $11,280 to $11, 520 (page 60).

- If you reach 65 in 1996 or 1997, the delayed retirement credit is 5% for each full year that you do not receive your benefits (page 55).

- Beginning with tax year 1994, taxes on Social Security benefits increase, making up to 85% subject to federal income taxes for high-income beneficiaries.

- The Medicare Part A deductible increases from $716 to $736. After 60 days in a hospital, you must pay $184 per day for 30 days, and then $368 per day for 60 "lifetime reserve" days (pages 106).

- The Medicare Part B monthly premium declines from $46.10 to $42.50 (page 109).

Changes in the 1996 benefit levels have the following results:

- The maximum monthly benefit for a person retiring in 1996 at age 65 is $1,248, compared to $1,199 for 1995 retirees at age 65.

- The average monthly benefit for a retired worker is $720 compared to $698 at the beginning of 1995.

- The average monthly benefit for a retired couple is $1,215 compared to $1,178 at the beginning of 1995.

- The average monthly benefit for a young widow with two eligible children is $1,407 compared to $1,365 at the beginning of 1995.

- The average monthly benefit for an aged widow without children is $680 compared to $656 at the beginning of 1995.

- The average monthly benefit for a disabled worker is $682 compared to $661 at the beginning of 1995.

How To Use This Book

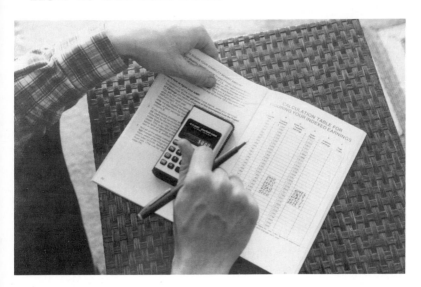

We've tried to make it easy. You can read through the whole book and get a clear overview of Social Security and Medicare, or you can turn to a specific section to get the answer to your question. Here's where to find the information you want:

What You Want To Know	Where To Find It
If you want to know about a specific **topic:**	Use the Table of Contents (pages 8-9). It lists each topic under every chapter.
To find approximate benefits in the event of:	See the Easy-Reference Tables on:

To calculate the benefit at:	See the calculation steps and tables on:

If you can't find an answer to your question, call the Social Security Administration at 800-772-1213. They're available to help. Social Security and Medicare **are** complicated subjects, but they are also important to you. It's worth a little of your time to learn something about them. Share this book with your family; then keep it handy as your permanent reference to SOCIAL SECURITY and MEDICARE.

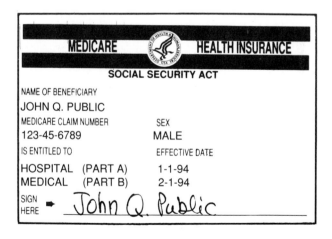

Contents

1

Who Is Covered

In this book, **worker** means anyone with earnings covered by Social Security. Almost everyone who is employed or self-employed is covered by Social Security and Medicare. The major **exceptions** are:

- Most federal government employees hired before 1984. They are covered by Medicare, but ordinarily not by Old-Age, Survivors, and Disability Insurance (Social Security). Instead, they are covered by Civil Service Retirement or a similar pension plan. Beginning in 1957, U.S. military personnel have been under Social Security.

- About 20% of state and local government employees. Each state and local government unit with a pension plan decides for itself whether to join Social Security; most have joined. Once elected, participation cannot be discontinued. After July 1, 1991, all state and local government employees who are not covered by a retirement plan of their employer are covered by Social Security and Medicare. All state and local government employees hired after March 1986 pay the 1.45% Medicare tax even if they do not have to pay the 6.2% Social Security tax.

- Railroad workers are covered under the separate, federally administered Railroad Retirement system. Workers with coverage under both Railroad Retirement and Social Security have their benefits coordinated.

2

Benefits Provided and Who Receives Them

Social Security pays benefits when you retire, become disabled, or die, if eligibility requirements are met.

Your spouse and children may also be eligible for benefits when you become entitled. The following information shows who most often receives Social Security cash benefits. Qualifications are different for each kind of benefit, as described later.

Monthly payments are increased each January to reflect changes in the cost of living.

When You Receive Social Security Benefits

Benefits normally arrive on the third day of the month after the month for which the benefit is paid. For example, you receive the benefit for February 1996 on March 3. If the third day of the month is a Saturday, Sunday, or holiday, benefits are delivered on the first business day before the third. The Social Security Administration recommends that you have your benefits directly deposited into your checking or savings account. The form required to arrange for a direct deposit can be obtained from your bank or other financial institution. Of course, you can ask to have checks mailed to you.

When You Retire Benefits May Be Paid To:

You
Age 62 or over

Your Spouse
Age 62 or over

Any age, if caring for your child who is under 16 or who is disabled before age 22

Your Unmarried Child
Under 18, or 18 if in high school, or any age if disabled before age 22

When You Become Disabled Benefits May Be Paid To:

You
Any age before Normal Retirement Age (page 47)

Your Spouse
Any age, if caring for your child who is under 16 or who is disabled before age 22

Age 62 or over

Your Unmarried Child
Under 18, or 18 if in high school, or any age if disabled before age 22

When You Die Benefits May Be Paid To:

Your Spouse
Any age, if caring for your child who is under 16 or who is disabled before age 22

Age 60 or over, or age 50-59 if disabled

Your Unmarried Child
Under 18, or 18 if in high school, or any age if disabled before age 22

3

What It Costs

Who Pays

You and your employer pay taxes for Social Security and Medicare. Your tax comes out of your pay. You and your employer each pay 6.2% for Social Security and 1.45% for Medicare Hospital Insurance. Your employer pays half the cost — you get all the benefits.

How Much

The taxes that you and your employer pay each year are based on:

- the tax rate (percent of pay) and
- the amount of your earnings taxed.

Current	Y-T-D	Deductions	Current	Y-T-D
$1,200.00	$27,600.00	FICA Tax Fed. Tax State Tax	$ 91.80 102.00 54.36	$2,111.40 2,346.00 1,250.28
$1,200.00	$27,600.00	Total Deductions	$248.16	$5,707.68

For Period Ending	NET PAY
11-12	$951.84

Two Taxes

Two separate payroll taxes are withheld from employees' wages:

> **Social Security:** This tax pays for monthly cash benefits to entitled beneficiaries.

> **Medicare (Hospital Insurance):** This tax pays for hospital benefits for people covered by Medicare when they become entitled.

For most purposes, the two taxes are simply added together and treated as one amount — hereinafter referred to as "payroll taxes." Self-employed persons (who are responsible for both the employer and employee taxes) report these taxes with their income tax returns.

You do not pay any Social Security tax on earnings over the **Maximum Taxable Amount.** In 1996, this amount is $62,700 for Social Security. There is no limit for Medicare.

Your Social Security tax equals:

The tax rate $\times$ Your earnings
(up to the Maximum Taxable Amount)

Your employer pays the same amount on your behalf.

Tax Rates are established by federal law.

The **Maximum Taxable Amount** for Social Security increases each year, based on increases in the average wages and salaries of all employees.

Example — Payroll Taxes

Suppose you earn $30,000 in 1996. How much tax will be paid?

	Tax Rate		Earnings		Amount of Tax
You, Social Security	6.20%	×	$30,000	=	$1,860.00
You, Medicare	1.45%	×	30,000	=	435.00
			Your Total		$2,295.00
Employer, Social Security	6.20%	×	$30,000	=	$1,860.00
Employer, Medicare	1.45%	×	30,000	=	435.00
			Employer Total		$2,295.00
			Grand Total		$4,590.00

Here's another example. Suppose you earn $100,000 in 1996.

	Tax Rate		Taxable Amount		Amount of Tax
You, Social Security	6.20%	×	$ 62,700	=	$ 3,887.40
You, Medicare	1.45%	×	100,000	=	1,450.00
			Total		$ 5,337.40
Employer, Social Security	6.20%	×	$ 62,700	=	$ 3,887.40
Employer, Medicare	1.45%	×	100,000	=	1,450.00
			Total		$ 5,337.40
			Grand Total		$10,674.80

Here is how the taxes have changed over the years:

Schedule of Social Security and Medicare Taxes

Years	Employee and Employer Tax Rate	Self-Employed Tax Rate	Maximum Earnings Taxed Annually
1937-49	1.00%	[a]	$ 3,000
1950	1.50	[a]	3,000
1951-53	1.50	2.25%	3,600
1954	2.00	3.00	3,600
1955-56	2.00	3.00	4,200
1957-58	2.25	3.375	4,200
1959	2.50	3.75	4,800
1960-61	3.00	4.50	4,800
1962	3.125	4.70	4,800
1963-65	3.625	5.40	4,800
1966	4.20	6.15	6,600
1967	4.40	6.40	6,600
1968	4.40	6.40	7,800
1969-70	4.80	6.90	7,800
1971	5.20	7.50	7,800
1972	5.20	7.50	9,000
1973	5.85	8.00	10,800
1974	5.85	7.90	13,200
1975	5.85	7.90	14,100
1976	5.85	7.90	15,300
1977	5.85	7.90	16,500
1978	6.05	8.10	17,700
1979	6.13	8.10	22,900
1980	6.13	8.10	25,900
1981	6.65	9.30	29,700
1982	6.70	9.35	32,400
1983	6.70	9.35	35,700
1984	6.70[b]	11.30	37,800
1985	7.05	11.80	39,600
1986	7.15	12.30	42,000
1987	7.15	12.30	43,800
1988	7.51	13.02	45,000
1989	7.51	13.02	48,000
1990	7.65	15.30[c]	51,300
1991	7.65	15.30[c]	53,400[d]
1992	7.65	15.30[c]	55,500[d]
1993	7.65	15.30[c]	57,600[d]
1994	7.65	15.30[c]	60,600[d]
1995	7.65	15.30[c]	61,200[d]
1996	7.65	15.30[c]	62,700[d]

[a] Self-employed persons were not covered until 1951.
[b] Employers paid 7.00% in 1984.
[c] Half the tax is deductible as a business expense for federal income taxes.
[d] This is the maximum for Social Security. This figure will rise in the future as the national average wage rises. The maximum for Medicare was $125,000 in 1991, $130,200 in 1992, and $135,000 in 1993; for 1994 and after, there is no limit.

The following table shows the total Social Security taxes (but not Medicare taxes) paid by an employee who retires at the normal retirement age of 65 at the beginning of various years. Earned income taxed for Social Security is assumed to have begun in the year that age 22 is reached. Three different earnings levels are shown.

Total Social Security Taxes
Paid by Employees[1] with Steady Work Records

| Age 65 in Year | If Your Earnings Were Equal To: | | |
	Maximum Taxable Amount or more	U.S. Average Earnings[2]	One-Half of U.S. Average Earnings
2000	$72,640	$32,555	$16,277
1999	68,149	30,742	15,371
1998	63,824	29,003	14,501
1997	59,674	27,331	13,666
1996	55,655	25,711	12,855
1995	51,821	24,165	12,082
1994	48,081	22,677	11,338
1993	44,369	21,242	10,621
1992	40,828	19,833	9,917
1991	37,417	18,435	9,217
1990	34,136	17,104	8,552
1989	30,985	15,819	7,910
1988	28,106	14,621	7,311
1987	25,409	13,468	6,734
1986	22,943	12,435	6,217
1985	20,579	11,462	5,731
1984	18,352	10,516	5,258
1983	16,340	9,657	4,828
1982	14,443	8,845	4,423
1981	12,723	8,071	4,036
1980	11,164	7,346	3,673
1979	9,848	6,710	3,355
1978	8,685	6,127	3,063
1977	7,791	5,594	2,797
1976	6,974	5,110	2,555
1975	6,217	4,653	2,326

[1] For 1990 and later, self-employed persons pay twice the amount that employees pay (but less than this before 1990).

[2] U.S. average earnings in 1995 is estimated to be $24,673; subsequent years are also estimates.

W-2 Form (Annual Earnings Report)

The W-2 form that you get from your employer shows the 6.2% Social Security tax separately from the 1.45% Medicare tax. This is because there is a maximum amount of earnings taxed for Social Security, but no maximum for Medicare (page 14).

a Control number 0001		Void ☐			
b Employer's identification number 13-2834414				1 Wages, tips, other compensation 75,000.00	2 Federal income tax withheld 9,175.00
c Employer's name, address, and ZIP code Grinstead Mfg. Co., Inc. 5701 Ringwood Drive Pittsburgh, Pennsylvania 15219				3 Social security wages 57,600.00	4 Social security tax withheld 3,571.20
				5 Medicare wages and tips 75,000.00	6 Medicare tax withheld 1,087.50
				7 Social security tips none	8 Allocated tips none
d Employee's social security number 123-45-6789				9 Advance EIC payment 0.00	10 Dependent care benefits none
e Employee's name, address, and ZIP code John Q. Public 1907 Garden Court Pittsburgh, Pennsylvania 15270				11 Nonqualified plans none	12 Benefits included in Box 1 430.20
				13	14 Other none
	15 Statutory employee ☐	Deceased ☐	Pension plan ☐	Legal rep ☐ 942 emp ☐ Subtotal ☐	Deferred compensation ☐
16 State Employer's state I.D. No. PA	17 State wages, tips, etc. 75,000.00	18 State income tax 2,840.00	19 Locality name Pittsburgh	20 Local wages, tips, etc. 75,000.00	21 Local income tax 1,132.00

Department of the Treasury—Internal Revenue Service

W-2 Wage and Tax Statement **1995**
Copy C For EMPLOYEE'S RECORDS (See Notice on back.)

Taxes Not Deductible

Social Security and Medicare taxes paid by employees are not deductible for federal income taxes.

What Is Taxed

All salaries, wages, bonuses, and commissions that you receive for working are taxed and credited to your earnings record. The Social Security tax is withheld until the Maximum Taxable Amount for the year is reached. The Medicare tax is withheld from **every** paycheck.

In addition to cash payments, taxable amounts include the value of clothing, meals, and lodging, except meals and lodging provided for the convenience of your employer. The first six months of sick pay are taxed. The cost of employer-provided group term life insurance coverage exceeding $50,000 is also taxed. Employee contributions to "cash-or-deferred" plans under IRC Section 401(k) are taxed, as are contributions to tax-deferred annuities under Section 403(b), even though federal income taxes on such amounts are deferred. This demonstrates that the rules for Social Security taxes and income taxes are not always the same.

If you have questions about what is taxable, call the IRS.

What Is Not Taxed

Payments from almost all employee benefit plans are excluded from payroll taxes, as are **employer** payments into such plans. Also, items of little value provided by your employer are generally not taxed. For example, you aren't taxed for using the company parking lot or medical clinic, or for discounts on company products. Contributions to a "flexible spending account" under IRC Section 125 are free of payroll and income taxes. Such plans permit an employee to authorize a salary reduction and use the money for such things as unreimbursed healthcare expenses and dependent care assistance.

Payroll Taxes on Non-Qualified Payments

Retired employees often receive a lump-sum payment, or a series of payments, outside of the qualified (IRS approved) retirement plan. These arrangements may be called deferred compensation plans, supplemental executive retirement programs (SERPs), severance payments, or some other name. The Social Security and Medicare tax rules for such payments are complicated, but here are some fundamentals. If the agreement includes a "substantial risk of forfeiture," such as a provision prohibiting competition, then the taxes apply as the payments are made.

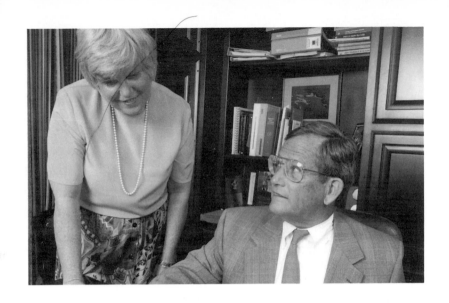

Where no "substantial risk of forfeiture" exists, then the tax is payable in the year that the right to the money becomes fixed or vested. This means that the present value of the future payments must be determined. The IRS has not issued final regulations on this, but it has been accepting employer determinations that are reasonable.

If the retiree has already paid the maximum tax for the year that the non-qualified benefit became vested, there is no need to make the calculation. But the problem has been complicated by the removal of the ceiling on the taxable wage base for the Medicare portion of the tax for years beginning with 1994. While many recipients of non-qualified payments will have had regular salary payments which exceeded the taxable wage base for Social Security ($62,700 in 1996) — they will still have to pay the 1.45% Medicare tax on the value of the non-qualified payment if the benefit became vested after 1993.

Director Fees

Special Social Security and Medicare tax rules apply to fees paid to members of corporate boards of directors. Such fees are classified as self-employment income.

Ordinarily, self-employment income is taxable for Social Security and Medicare and counts against the Earnings Limitation when you receive it. However, for corporate directors the law is slightly different. Director fees count against the Earnings Limitation when they are earned, even if the director chooses to defer payment until later. This means a director cannot collect Social Security benefits while **earning** substantial fees. In 1988-90, Social Security and Medicare taxes were also paid on deferred director fees when earned, but starting in 1991 taxes have been payable on director fees **when received.**

Domestic Service

Beginning with 1994, wages of $1,000 or more per year paid to workers 18 and over to work in or around an employer's home are subject to Social Security and Medicare payroll taxes. Only payments in money are subject to these taxes for this type of work — not material things such as meals or clothing. The law exempts such household workers under 18 who are students, or if they have another occupation which is their principal one.

Agricultural Labor

If you are paid $150 or more in a calendar year from one employer for farm work or if that employer pays at least $2,500 to all employees for such labor during the year, you are generally subject to the payroll taxes, and your earnings will count in figuring your benefits.

Tips
If you receive tips of $20 or more in a month, all of your cash tips are treated as regular wages.

Two or More Employers
If you work for more than one employer, **each one** must withhold Medicare taxes on all of your earnings, and up to the Maximum Taxable Amount for Social Security. If your **total earnings** from all employers are more than the Maximum Taxable Amount, then you will have paid too much tax.

What happens when you overpay? You can credit the overpayment against the federal income taxes that you owe when you file your return, or you can claim a refund (page 177). Your employers do not get a credit or refund for their payments.

Family Employment
If you are self-employed and hire your spouse, parent, or child age 18 or older **in the course of your business,** this is covered employment. If employment is not in the course of your business, this is **not** covered.

Benefits for the Self-Employed

If you are self-employed, you are probably covered by Social Security and Medicare.

As a self-employed person, you are entitled to a deduction in computing net earnings to reflect the fact that employees do not pay FICA taxes on the value of the **employer's** FICA tax. Accordingly, you deduct from net earnings from self-employment, an amount equal to one-half of the self-employment tax on such earnings, at a rate of 15.3%. This means that you pay the tax on 92.35% of your net annual income from self-employment (if the result is at least $400), which amount is considered as your self-employment income for benefit purposes. In general, net income is figured under the same rules as for income tax purposes. You determine your payroll taxes on self-employment income using a special income tax form (Schedule SE). Also, you deduct half of your Social Security and Medicare self-employment tax as a business expense on your income tax return.

If you are in more than one type of self-employment, the profits and losses of all businesses are added together to figure your net income.

If you are both self-employed and an employee, you pay taxes on your employee earnings at the employee tax rate. If you earn the Maximum Taxable Amount for Social Security (or more) as an employee, you do not pay any Social Security self-employment tax. If you earn less than such Maximum Taxable Amount as an employee, then you must pay the Social Security self-employment tax on the amount of your self-employment earnings (after adjustment by the 92.35% factor) that brings you up to the Maximum Taxable Amount, when added to your wages as an employee. With respect to the separate Medicare tax, you pay it on **all** of your earnings as an employee, and in self-employment (page 14) after the 92.35% adjustment.

You must pay the Social Security tax even if you don't have to pay any federal income tax. If a husband and wife file a joint return, each one who has any self-employment income must file his or her own Schedule SE.

The Tax Rates and Maximum Taxable Amounts for the self-employed are shown on page 16.

Benefits for the Self Employed
Benefits for the self employed are the same as for employees.

Taxes after Benefits Begin

If you work while receiving benefits, you still pay Social Security and Medicare taxes on your earnings.

Social Security benefits may be reduced if earned income exceeds the Earnings Limitation (see pages 60-64).

Although Social Security benefits are tax-free for most people, those with high total incomes must include up to 85% of their benefits for federal income tax purposes. There are two step-rate thresholds for single persons, $25,000 and $34,000. For married persons, the thresholds are $32,000 and $44,000 if they file a joint return. Married couples filing separate returns who live together at any time during the year have zero thresholds (if not so living together, they are considered as single persons).

The Preliminary Adjusted Gross Income (earnings, pensions, dividends and taxable interest from investments, and other sources), plus interest on tax-exempt bonds, plus 50% of Social Security benefits, is compared with the thresholds. Then, 50% of any excess over the first threshold, plus 35% of any excess over the second threshold is included in Adjusted Gross Income. Such amount, however, cannot exceed the smaller of (a) 85% of the benefits or (b) 50% of the benefits, plus 85% of any excess over the second threshold.

Examples of Federal Income Taxes on Social Security Benefits

Single Person with $10,000/Year in Benefits

Preliminary Adjusted Gross Income (PAGI) $31,000
Tax-free bond interest   2,000
50% of Social Security benefit ($10,000)   5,000
Modified Adjusted Gross Income (MAGI) $38,000

Excess of MAGI over first threshold ($25,000) $13,000
Excess of MAGI over second threshold
($34,000) . . . . $ 4,000

(1) 50% of MAGI over 1st threshold, plus 35% of
   MAGI over 2nd threshold
   (.50 × $13,000 + .35 × $4,000) . . . . $ 7,900
(2) 85% of benefits (.85 × $10,000) . . . . $ 8,500
(3) 50% of benefits, plus 85% of MAGI over 2nd
   threshold (.50 × $10,000 + .85 × $4,000) . . . . $ 8,400

Thus, the smallest of these three figures, $7,900, is added to the
PAGI of $31,000, making the Adjusted Gross Income $38,900.

Married Couple with $20,000/Year in Benefits

Preliminary Adjusted Gross Income (PAGI) $50,000
Tax-free bond interest   4,000
50% of Social Security benefits ($20,000) 10,000
Modified Adjusted Gross Income (MAGI) $64,000

Excess of MAGI over first threshold ($32,000) $32,000
Excess of MAGI over second threshold
($44,000) $20,000

(1) 50% of MAGI over 1st threshold, plus 35% of
   MAGI over 2nd threshold
   (.50 × $32,000 + .35 × $20,000) $23,000
(2) 85% of benefits (.85 × $20,000) $17,000
(3) 50% of benefits, plus 85% of MAGI over 2nd
   threshold (.50 × $20,000 + .85 × $20,000) $27,000

Thus, the smallest of these three figures, $17,000, is added to the
PAGI of $50,000, making the Adjusted Gross Income $67,000.

Most states do not tax Social Security benefits, but you should
consult your tax advisor.

4

Retirement Benefits

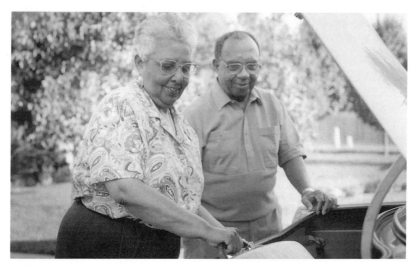

All monthly benefits are based on your **Primary Insurance Amount** (PIA) which is the amount you would receive if you retired at your Normal Retirement Age (NRA), currently age 65. (For persons born after 1937, the NRA will gradually increase, see page 47.)

The formula for calculating your PIA is described on page 151.

Easy-Reference Table

The table on the next page shows the approximate amount of the age-65 monthly benefits for you and your spouse. We assume that you have worked steadily and received pay raises at a rate equal to the U.S. average throughout your working career. In addition, we assume that your earnings and the general level of wages and salaries in the country will stay the same until you retire. This way, the table shows the value of your benefits in today's dollars.

Monthly Benefits at Age 65

Your Age in 1996	Who Receives Benefits	Your Present Annual Earnings				
		$15,000	**$24,000**	**$36,000**	**$48,000**	**$62,700 and Up**
65	You	$622	$845	$1,100	$1,179	$1,248
	Spouse	311	422	550	589	624
64	You	637	865	1,128	1,213	1,289
	Spouse	318	432	564	606	644
63	You	626	850	1,110	1,197	1,277
	Spouse	313	425	555	598	638
62	You	626	850	1,111	1,203	1,287
	Spouse	313	425	555	601	643
61	You	627	851	1,114	1,210	1,299
	Spouse	313	425	557	605	649
55*	You	604	821	1,077	1,193	1,308
	Spouse	298	406	532	589	646
50*	You	594	809	1,057	1,186	1,323
	Spouse	291	397	519	582	650
45*	You	598	815	1,061	1,197	1,356
	Spouse	293	400	521	587	666
40*	You	587	802	1,040	1,174	1,338
	Spouse	286	391	507	572	652
35*	You	562	768	994	1,122	1,281
	Spouse	270	369	477	539	616
30*	You	566	774	997	1,127	1,287
	Spouse	272	372	479	542	618

*These amounts are reduced for retirement at age 65 because the NRA is higher for these persons (see pages 49-50 and 153).

Starting with the year you turn 62, your benefits are increased to reflect changes in the cost of living, whether or not you are retired. These increases are effective every December and are ordinarily payable to beneficiaries beginning in January. They are included in the table for persons who became age 62 before 1996. No cost-of-living increases are included for December 1996 or later.

There is a **Maximum Family Benefit** that generally applies when more than two beneficiaries are entitled to payments on the same Social Security earnings record (pages 59-60).

This table shows only **approximate** retirement benefits. For a more accurate figure, you can follow the steps on pages 35-46. For an exact figure, you need your entire earnings history, which you can obtain by completing and mailing Form SSA-7004 in the back of this book.

Benefits as a Percentage of Pay

The table on page 27 gives you a close estimate of your age-65 benefit in today's dollars. Inflation would cause the actual dollars to be much higher, however. The graph on page 29 illustrates the benefit at Normal Retirement Age as a percentage of pay **subject to the Social Security tax** in the year before you retire. It applies to anyone who has had **steady** earnings.

First, find your annual pay on the graph. For example, if you earn $35,000, you find it on the bottom (horizontal) line of the chart. Reading up to the graph line and over to the vertical line on the left side reveals that you could expect a benefit of 37.2% of your final level of pay. If no future inflation occurs, your annual benefit would be $13,020 per year (37.2% × $35,000).

If your earnings are equal to the U.S. average (currently, about $25,000), you can expect to receive a benefit of about 41% of pay. If you always had the maximum taxable earnings, you can expect to receive about 25% of that **portion** of your pay subject to the Social Security tax (gradually increasing to 27½% during the next 20 years). The **replacement ratio** refers to the percentage of your pay that is replaced by your Social Security retirement benefit.

Social Security Replacement Ratios

(For retirement at Normal Retirement Age — 65 until 2003, then gradually increasing to 67 after 2026)

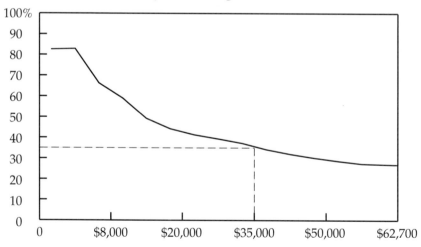

Annual Earnings in Year Before Retirement

Qualifications for Retirement Benefits

To qualify for retirement benefits, you must be **fully insured;** that is, you must have the required number of **credits** under Social Security. Most workers need 40 credits to qualify for retirement benefits — or about 10 years of work. Workers born before 1929 need fewer credits.

Through 1977, you earned one credit for any calendar quarter in which you had wages or salary of at least $50 in covered employment. Since 1978, you earn credits on the basis of your annual earnings, up to four credits in any year. In 1996, one credit is recorded for every $640 you earn during the year, with four credits if you earn $2,560 or more. (The amounts required to earn a credit in 1978-95 are shown in column G of the worksheet on page 38.)

The table below shows how many credits you need to be fully insured. If you were born on January 1, refer to the year prior to the year of your birth.

Credits Required To Qualify for Retirement Benefits

Year of Birth	Credits
1926	37
1927	38
1928	39
After 1928	40

Applying for Benefits

If you think you are eligible for benefits, you should file an application. It is better to apply for benefits and be denied than not to apply for benefits to which you are entitled. It's also important to apply on time, because there are strict limits on retroactive benefits. (See pages 32-34 for a detailed discussion of when to apply for retirement benefits.)

You can apply for Social Security benefits by telephone or in person at a local office. You can call Social Security at 800-772-1213 and schedule an appointment either for a telephone application or a personal interview; they will advise you what documents you need. Social Security will need original or certified copies of documents. They will make their own photocopies and return all documents to you.

Almost all applicants will need to present a birth certificate. In the rare case where a birth certificate is not available, Social Security will advise what alternative documents can be submitted. You should know your own Social Security number and the number of your spouse.

When To Apply for Social Security Benefits

The Social Security Administration advises people to file claims about three months before they want the benefits to begin, but it does not always recommend what month is best for the claimant's first effective month. This section will address that issue, especially as to how it has been affected by legislative changes that occurred in 1990.

First, there is the question of retroactivity of benefits when they are not filed for in a timely manner. For years, only 12 months of retroactivity was allowed. This limit was instituted on the grounds that, if a person did not file for Social Security benefits within a reasonable time, then they were not really "needed."

Several years ago, the 12-month limit was reduced to 6 months for all but disability benefits. Also, it was provided that such retroactivity could not result in **permanently** reducing the benefit. **Temporarily** reduced benefits were permitted. For example, this meant that one could apply retroactively for up to six months providing no benefits were actually paid because of the Social Security earnings limitation (pages 60-64). The Omnibus Budget Reconciliation Act (OBRA) of 1990 eliminated the right to file for non-disability benefits retroactively as to benefits before age 65. In some cases, this caused a large disparity in benefit amounts for two claims which were identical except for the application date.

For example, Mr. Anderson and Mr. Thomas (who have no eligible dependents) have both earned at least the maximum amount taxed by Social Security each year since 1951. Their Primary Insurance Amounts (PIAs), payable at age 65 in 1996, are $1,250 per month. Prior to attaining age 65 in July 1996, they had reduced their work loads some, but each had earned $28,200 to date. They both reduced their work hours further, but earn $970 per month for the rest of the year starting in July.

Mr. Anderson applied for Social Security retirement benefits in July, effective for that month. Because his earnings each month for the balance of the year exceed the permissible amount of $960 under the Social Security monthly earnings limitation, he cannot receive benefits under this test (page 60). Neither can he collect any benefits for 1996 when he uses the annual earnings test, demonstrated as follows:

Earnings, first 6 months	$28,200	
Earnings, second 6 months	5,820	(6 mos. × $970/mo.)
Total	$34,020	
Permissible earnings	11,520	
Excess earnings	$22,500	
Potential loss of benefits	$ 7,500	(one-third)
Benefit amount, second 6 months	$ 7,500	(6 mos. × $1,250/mo.)

Mr. Thomas on the other hand, applies for benefits in January, with the effective date that month even though he also intends to work through June. His benefit is reduced slightly from his PIA of $1,250 because of claiming it six months before the Normal Retirement Age. The reduction is 3.33%, making the benefit $1,208 ($1,250 × .9667). He **cannot** use the monthly earnings test either because of exceeding the permissible earnings of $960 in each month of the year. He **can** use the annual earnings test to his advantage, however, as follows:

Earnings, first 6 months	$28,200	
Earnings, second 6 months	5,820	(6 mos. × $970/mo.)
Total	$34,020	
Permissible earnings	11,520	
Excess earnings	$22,500	
Potential loss of benefits	$ 7,500	(one-third)
Benefit (January-June)	$ 7,250	(6 mos. × $1,208/mo.)
Difference	$ 250	(benefit loss for July)

Because all benefits payable for months before attaining age 65 have been withheld, the benefit amount is recomputed and increased to the unreduced $1,250. Now, the remaining $250 of benefits to be withheld is met by paying Mr. Thomas $1,000 for July ($1,250 — $250). Combined with $6,250 (5 mos. × $1,250) for the balance of the year, his total benefits are $7,250 greater than Mr. Anderson — simply by applying earlier. If he had a wife or other family members who were entitled to benefits on his work record, the difference in benefits could be much larger. In the case of Mr. Anderson, there would be a small compensating offset for the loss of $7,250 in benefits. This would occur because a Delayed Retirement Credit (page 55) for six months (July - December) would later be payable, for life, on his benefits at a rate of 2.5% ($^{6}/_{12}$ × 5%).

This provision should be repealed. However, if it is not, new beneficiaries who expect to have significant earned income after retirement should apply in January of the year in which they plan to commence benefits, just to be safe. However, if you plan to apply for benefits in the year in which you attain the minimum age to qualify (age 62), you cannot apply more than four months before attaining that age.

For persons who attain age 66-69 in a particular year during which they plan to "retire," the best strategy is to file the claim effective for no later than July. Under these circumstances, full retroactivity to the start of the year would be possible. The law permits retroactivity in these cases because, in doing this, there is no reduction in benefits. Similarly, persons who attain age 70 in a particular year and are still working, should file a claim effective for at least the month of becoming 70. In any event, for persons of any age beyond 65, filing a claim effective for January would not be a disadvantage.

How To Figure Your Retirement Benefit Amount

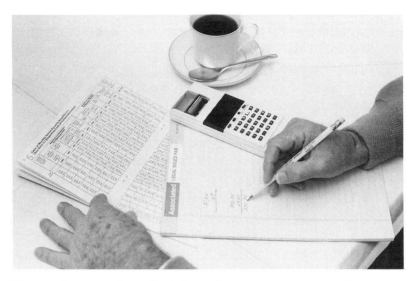

Your retirement benefit is based on your Primary Insurance Amount (PIA). To figure your PIA, you need to know your Average Indexed Monthly Earnings (AIME), which is based on your lifetime earnings history. If you were born in 1934 or later, you can figure your own AIME by following the steps below and using the worksheet on page 38. If you were born before 1934, use the appropriate worksheet that follows (see pages 39-46). (If you were born on January 1, refer to the year prior to the year of your birth.) This will enable you to make a good estimate of your PIA. Of course, to get a completely accurate PIA, you need your entire earnings history right up to the time of your retirement.

The PIA is the amount payable to you at your Normal Retirement Age, which is 65 for persons born before 1938. If you retire earlier, your benefit will be less than the PIA (pages 48-55). If you retire later, it will be more than the PIA (pages 55-56).

Here's how to figure your AIME:

(1) In column C of the worksheet for your year of birth, enter your earnings for each year after 1950. **You can get this information from the Earnings and Benefit Estimate Statement** that you can request from the Social Security Administration (page 176). If your earnings for any year were more than the Maximum Taxable Amount, use the Maximum Taxable Amount.

(2) Now enter in the last two lines of column C your expected earnings for 1996 and for all **future** years that you plan to work after 1996. For this purpose you should assume future earnings to be the same as 1996, so that your benefit will be more closely related to the value of today's dollar. Remember that higher earnings resulting from the increase in the cost of living will be balanced by higher costs generally. If you are 62 in 1996 or earlier, do not consider earnings after 1995 when figuring the benefit payable in 1996.

(3) Now multiply the earnings for all years by the Index Factors in column D. The index factors make past earnings comparable to the level of earnings today. Enter the results of your multiplication in column E, Indexed Earnings.

(4) Not all indexed earnings are used to figure your AIME. The table on page 37 shows how many years of earnings to use. If you were born on January 1, refer to the year prior to the year of your birth. (The rule for determining the number of years to use is on page 150.) Enter the number of years you must use _____

(5) On the worksheet, put a check mark in column F, High Years, by the years of your highest indexed earnings in column E until you have checked the number of years you must use from (4). For the "1997+" box, write the number of years that it represents, if this is a high year.

(6) Add up all the indexed earnings in column E for the years you have checked in column F. (If the "1997+" line is to be used, multiply the number in column F by the earnings in column E and use the result in the addition.)

.... $ _____

(7) Multiply the number of years in (4) by 12 to get months.

.... _____

(8) Divide the total earnings shown in (6) by the months shown in (7) to get your AIME (drop cents). $ _____

Now, to figure your PIA:

(9) If you were born in 1934, or later, look at the table on pages 84-85. Find the number in the first column that is closest to your AIME. The numbers on this line are your approximate PIA and the other benefits based on it. For a more precise benefit determination, apply the 1996 benefit formula shown on page 151. The benefit amount is increased by the cost-of-living percentage effective for December of the year in which you reach age 62 and for all subsequent years, whether or not you have actually retired.

If you were born in 1924-1933, use the benefit formula for your age shown on page 151.

Number of Years Used To Figure
Average Indexed Monthly Earnings

Year of Birth	Number of Years
1926	32
1927	33
1928	34
After 1928	35

Worksheet for Figuring Indexed Earnings *only* if Born in **1934** or later

A Calendar Year	B Maximum Taxable Amount	C Enter Your Taxable Earnings ×	D Index Factor =	E Indexed Earnings	F High Years	G Earnings Required for a Credit
1951	$ 3,600		8.48595			$ 50
1952	3,600		7.98889			50
1953	3,600		7.56617			50
1954	3,600		7.52733			50
1955	4,200		7.19490			50
1956	4,200		6.72455			50
1957	4,200		6.52261			50
1958	4,200		6.46566			50
1959	4,800		6.16047			50
1960	4,800		5.92783			50
1961	4,800		5.81231			50
1962	4,800		5.53515			50
1963	4,800		5.40266			50
1964	4,800		5.19053			50
1965	4,800		5.09872			50
1966	6,600		4.81000			50
1967	6,600		4.55621			50
1968	7,800		4.26320			50
1969	7,800		4.03028			50
1970	7,800		3.83974			50
1971	7,800		3.65603			50
1972	9,000		3.32972			50
1973	10,800		3.13364			50
1974	13,200		2.95782			50
1975	14,100		2.75214			50
1976	15,300		2.57450			50
1977	16,500		2.42893			50
1978	17,700		2.25023			250
1979	22,900		2.06922			260
1980	25,900		1.89824			290
1981	29,700		1.72463			310
1982	32,400		1.63464			340
1983	35,700		1.55871			370
1984	37,800		1.47217			390
1985	39,600		1.41201			410
1986	42,000		1.37131			440
1987	43,800		1.28910			460
1988	45,000		1.22859			470
1989	48,000		1.18179			500
1990	51,300		1.12962			520
1991	53,400		1.08903			540
1992	55,500		1.03567			570
1993	57,600		1.02684			590
1994	60,600		1.00000			620
1995	61,200		1.00000			630
1996	62,700		1.00000			640
1997+	*		1.00000			*

*To be determined (see page 14 as to column B and page 30 as to column G).
Note: Index factors change each year based on U.S. average wage.

Worksheet for Figuring Your Indexed Earnings *only* if Born in **1933**

A Calendar Year	B Maximum Taxable Amount	C Enter Your Taxable Earnings	×	D Index Factor	=	E Indexed Earnings	F High Years
1951	$ 3,600			8.26415			
1952	3,600			7.78008			
1953	3,600			7.36841			
1954	3,600			7.33058			
1955	4,200			7.00684			
1956	4,200			6.54879			
1957	4,200			6.35213			
1958	4,200			6.29666			
1959	4,800			5.99945			
1960	4,800			5.77289			
1961	4,800			5.66039			
1962	4,800			5.39047			
1963	4,800			5.26144			
1964	4,800			5.05486			
1965	4,800			4.96546			
1966	6,600			4.68428			
1967	6,600			4.43712			
1968	7,800			4.15177			
1969	7,800			3.92494			
1970	7,800			3.73937			
1971	7,800			3.56047			
1972	9,000			3.24269			
1973	10,800			3.05174			
1974	13,200			2.88051			
1975	14,100			2.68021			
1976	15,300			2.50720			
1977	16,500			2.36544			
1978	17,700			2.19142			
1979	22,900			2.01514			
1980	25,900			1.84862			
1981	29,700			1.67955			
1982	32,400			1.59192			
1983	35,700			1.51797			
1984	37,800			1.43369			
1985	39,600			1.37510			
1986	42,000			1.33546			
1987	43,800			1.25540			
1988	45,000			1.19647			
1989	48,000			1.15090			
1990	51,300			1.10009			
1991	53,400			1.06057			
1992	55,500			1.00860			
1993	57,600			1.00000			
1994	60,600			1.00000			
1995	61,200			1.00000			
1996	62,700			1.00000			
1997+	*			1.00000			

*To be determined.

Worksheet for Figuring Your Indexed Earnings *only* if Born in **1932**

A Calendar Year	B Maximum Taxable Amount	C Enter Your Taxable Earnings	×	D Index Factor	=	E Indexed Earnings	F High Years
1951	$ 3,600			8.19368			
1952	3,600			7.71374			
1953	3,600			7.30558			
1954	3,600			7.26807			
1955	4,200			6.94710			
1956	4,200			6.49295			
1957	4,200			6.29796			
1958	4,200			6.24297			
1959	4,800			5.94829			
1960	4,800			5.72367			
1961	4,800			5.61213			
1962	4,800			5.34451			
1963	4,800			5.21658			
1964	4,800			5.01176			
1965	4,800			4.92312			
1966	6,600			4.64434			
1967	6,600			4.39929			
1968	7,800			4.11637			
1969	7,800			3.89148			
1970	7,800			3.70749			
1971	7,800			3.53011			
1972	9,000			3.21504			
1973	10,800			3.02572			
1974	13,200			2.85595			
1975	14,100			2.65736			
1976	15,300			2.48583			
1977	16,500			2.34527			
1978	17,700			2.17273			
1979	22,900			1.99795			
1980	25,900			1.83286			
1981	29,700			1.66523			
1982	32,400			1.57834			
1983	35,700			1.50502			
1984	37,800			1.42146			
1985	39,600			1.36338			
1986	42,000			1.32408			
1987	43,800			1.24470			
1988	45,000			1.18627			
1989	48,000			1.14109			
1990	51,300			1.09071			
1991	53,400			1.05152			
1992	55,500			1.00000			
1993	57,600			1.00000			
1994	60,600			1.00000			
1995	61,200			1.00000			
1996	62,700			1.00000			
1997+	*			1.00000			

*To be determined.

Worksheet for Figuring Your Indexed Earnings *only* if Born in **1931**

A	B	C		D		E	F
Calendar Year	Maximum Taxable Amount	Enter Your Taxable Earnings	×	Index Factor	=	Indexed Earnings	High Years
1951	$ 3,600			7.79219			
1952	3,600			7.33577			
1953	3,600			6.94761			
1954	3,600			6.91194			
1955	4,200			6.60669			
1956	4,200			6.17480			
1957	4,200			5.98937			
1958	4,200			5.93707			
1959	4,800			5.65683			
1960	4,800			5.44321			
1961	4,800			5.33714			
1962	4,800			5.08263			
1963	4,800			4.96097			
1964	4,800			4.76619			
1965	4,800			4.68189			
1966	6,600			4.41677			
1967	6,600			4.18373			
1968	7,800			3.91467			
1969	7,800			3.70080			
1970	7,800			3.52583			
1971	7,800			3.35714			
1972	9,000			3.05750			
1973	10,800			2.87746			
1974	13,200			2.71601			
1975	14,100			2.52715			
1976	15,300			2.36402			
1977	16,500			2.23035			
1978	17,700			2.06627			
1979	22,900			1.90005			
1980	25,900			1.74305			
1981	29,700			1.58364			
1982	32,400			1.50100			
1983	35,700			1.43128			
1984	37,800			1.35181			
1985	39,600			1.29657			
1986	42,000			1.25920			
1987	43,800			1.18371			
1988	45,000			1.12814			
1989	48,000			1.08518			
1990	51,300			1.03727			
1991	53,400			1.00000			
1992	55,500			1.00000			
1993	57,600			1.00000			
1994	60,600			1.00000			
1995	61,200			1.00000			
1996	62,700			1.00000			
1997+	*			1.00000			

*To be determined.

Worksheet for Figuring Your Indexed Earnings *only* if Born in **1930**

A Calendar Year	B Maximum Taxable Amount	C Enter Your Taxable Earnings	×	D Index Factor	=	E Indexed Earnings	F High Years
1951	$ 3,600			7.51225			
1952	3,600			7.07222			
1953	3,600			6.69800			
1954	3,600			6.66362			
1955	4,200			6.36934			
1956	4,200			5.95295			
1957	4,200			5.77419			
1958	4,200			5.72377			
1959	4,800			5.45360			
1960	4,800			5.24765			
1961	4,800			5.14539			
1962	4,800			4.90003			
1963	4,800			4.78274			
1964	4,800			4.59495			
1965	4,800			4.51368			
1966	6,600			4.25809			
1967	6,600			4.03342			
1968	7,800			3.77403			
1969	7,800			3.56784			
1970	7,800			3.39915			
1971	7,800			3.23653			
1972	9,000			2.94765			
1973	10,800			2.77408			
1974	13,200			2.61843			
1975	14,100			2.43635			
1976	15,300			2.27909			
1977	16,500			2.15022			
1978	17,700			1.99203			
1979	22,900			1.83179			
1980	25,900			1.68043			
1981	29,700			1.52674			
1982	32,400			1.44708			
1983	35,700			1.37986			
1984	37,800			1.30325			
1985	39,600			1.24999			
1986	42,000			1.21396			
1987	43,800			1.14118			
1988	45,000			1.08761			
1989	48,000			1.04619			
1990	51,300			1.00000			
1991	53,400			1.00000			
1992	55,500			1.00000			
1993	57,600			1.00000			
1994	60,600			1.00000			
1995	61,200			1.00000			
1996	62,700			1.00000			
1997+	*			1.00000			

*To be determined.

Worksheet for Figuring Your Indexed Earnings *only* if Born in **1929**

A Calendar Year	B Maximum Taxable Amount	C Enter Your Taxable Earnings	×	D Index Factor	=	E Indexed Earnings	F High Years
1951	$ 3,600			7.18056			
1952	3,600			6.75997			
1953	3,600			6.40227			
1954	3,600			6.36941			
1955	4,200			6.08812			
1956	4,200			5.69012			
1957	4,200			5.51925			
1958	4,200			5.47105			
1959	4,800			5.21281			
1960	4,800			5.01596			
1961	4,800			4.91821			
1962	4,800			4.68368			
1963	4,800			4.57157			
1964	4,800			4.39208			
1965	4,800			4.31439			
1966	6,600			4.07009			
1967	6,600			3.85533			
1968	7,800			3.60740			
1969	7,800			3.41031			
1970	7,800			3.24907			
1971	7,800			3.09363			
1972	9,000			2.81751			
1973	10,800			2.65160			
1974	13,200			2.50282			
1975	14,100			2.32878			
1976	15,300			2.17846			
1977	16,500			2.05529			
1978	17,700			1.90408			
1979	22,900			1.75091			
1980	25,900			1.60623			
1981	29,700			1.45933			
1982	32,400			1.38319			
1983	35,700			1.31893			
1984	37,800			1.24571			
1985	39,600			1.19480			
1986	42,000			1.16036			
1987	43,800			1.09080			
1988	45,000			1.03959			
1989	48,000			1.00000			
1990	51,300			1.00000			
1991	53,400			1.00000			
1992	55,500			1.00000			
1993	57,600			1.00000			
1994	60,600			1.00000			
1995	61,200			1.00000			
1996	62,700			1.00000			
1997+	*			1.00000			

*To be determined.

Worksheet for Figuring Your Indexed Earnings *only* if Born in **1928**

A Calendar Year	B Maximum Taxable Amount	C Enter Your Taxable Earnings	×	D Index Factor	=	E Indexed Earnings	F High Years
1951	$ 3,600			6.90709			
1952	3,600			6.50251			
1953	3,600			6.15844			
1954	3,600			6.12682			
1955	4,200			5.85624			
1956	4,200			5.47341			
1957	4,200			5.30904			
1958	4,200			5.26268			
1959	4,800			5.01427			
1960	4,800			4.82492			
1961	4,800			4.73090			
1962	4,800			4.50530			
1963	4,800			4.39746			
1964	4,800			4.22480			
1965	4,800			4.15008			
1966	6,600			3.91507			
1967	6,600			3.70850			
1968	7,800			3.47001			
1969	7,800			3.28043			
1970	7,800			3.12533			
1971	7,800			2.97580			
1972	9,000			2.71020			
1973	10,800			2.55061			
1974	13,200			2.40750			
1975	14,100			2.24009			
1976	15,300			2.09549			
1977	16,500			1.97701			
1978	17,700			1.83156			
1979	22,900			1.68423			
1980	25,900			1.54506			
1981	29,700			1.40375			
1982	32,400			1.33051			
1983	35,700			1.26870			
1984	37,800			1.19826			
1985	39,600			1.14930			
1986	42,000			1.11617			
1987	43,800			1.04925			
1988	45,000			1.00000			
1989	48,000			1.00000			
1990	51,300			1.00000			
1991	53,400			1.00000			
1992	55,500			1.00000			
1993	57,600			1.00000			
1994	60,600			1.00000			
1995	61,200			1.00000			
1996	62,700			1.00000			
1997+	*			1.00000			

*To be determined.

Worksheet for Figuring Your Indexed Earnings *only* if Born in 1927

A Calendar Year	B Maximum Taxable Amount	C Enter Your Taxable Earnings	×	D Index Factor	=	E Indexed Earnings	F High Years
1951	$ 3,600			6.58287			
1952	3,600			6.19728			
1953	3,600			5.86936			
1954	3,600			5.83923			
1955	4,200			5.58136			
1956	4,200			5.21649			
1957	4,200			5.05984			
1958	4,200			5.01565			
1959	4,800			4.77891			
1960	4,800			4.59844			
1961	4,800			4.50883			
1962	4,800			4.29382			
1963	4,800			4.19104			
1964	4,800			4.02649			
1965	4,800			3.95527			
1966	6,600			3.73130			
1967	6,600			3.53442			
1968	7,800			3.30713			
1969	7,800			3.12644			
1970	7,800			2.97863			
1971	7,800			2.83612			
1972	9,000			2.58299			
1973	10,800			2.43089			
1974	13,200			2.29449			
1975	14,100			2.13494			
1976	15,300			1.99713			
1977	16,500			1.88421			
1978	17,700			1.74559			
1979	22,900			1.60517			
1980	25,900			1.47254			
1981	29,700			1.33786			
1982	32,400			1.26805			
1983	35,700			1.20915			
1984	37,800			1.14202			
1985	39,600			1.09535			
1986	42,000			1.06377			
1987	43,800			1.00000			
1988	45,000			1.00000			
1989	48,000			1.00000			
1990	51,300			1.00000			
1991	53,400			1.00000			
1992	55,500			1.00000			
1993	57,600			1.00000			
1994	60,600			1.00000			
1995	61,200			1.00000			
1996	62,700			1.00000			
1997+	*			1.00000			

*To be determined.

Worksheet for Figuring Your Indexed Earnings *only* if Born in **1926**

A Calendar Year	B Maximum Taxable Amount	C Enter Your Taxable Earnings		D Index Factor		E Indexed Earnings	F High Years
1951	$ 3,600		×	6.18822	=		
1952	3,600			5.82575			
1953	3,600			5.51749			
1954	3,600			5.48916			
1955	4,200			5.24675			
1956	4,200			4.90375			
1957	4,200			4.75649			
1958	4,200			4.71496			
1959	4,800			4.49241			
1960	4,800			4.32276			
1961	4,800			4.23852			
1962	4,800			4.03640			
1963	4,800			3.93979			
1964	4,800			3.78510			
1965	4,800			3.71815			
1966	6,600			3.50761			
1967	6,600			3.32253			
1968	7,800			3.10886			
1969	7,800			2.93901			
1970	7,800			2.80006			
1971	7,800			2.66609			
1972	9,000			2.42813			
1973	10,800			2.28515			
1974	13,200			2.15693			
1975	14,100			2.00695			
1976	15,300			1.87740			
1977	16,500			1.77125			
1978	17,700			1.64094			
1979	22,900			1.50894			
1980	25,900			1.38426			
1981	29,700			1.25766			
1982	32,400			1.19203			
1983	35,700			1.13666			
1984	37,800			1.07355			
1985	39,600			1.02968			
1986	42,000			1.00000			
1987	43,800			1.00000			
1988	45,000			1.00000			
1989	48,000			1.00000			
1990	51,300			1.00000			
1991	53,400			1.00000			
1992	55,500			1.00000			
1993	57,600			1.00000			
1994	60,600			1.00000			
1995	61,200			1.00000			
1996	62,700			1.00000			
1997+	*			1.00000			

*To be determined.

Normal Retirement Age

Beginning with persons born in 1938, the Normal Retirement Age will gradually increase from age 65, eventually reaching age 67 for persons born after 1959. The benefit at the Normal Retirement Age is the Primary Insurance Amount (page 26).

The following table illustrates this important change:

Normal Retirement Age for Retired Worker and Spouses' Benefits	Year of Birth	Normal Retirement Age for Surviving Spouses' Benefits
65	Before 1938	65
65 and 2 months	1938	65
65 and 4 months	1939	65
65 and 6 months	1940	65 and 2 months
65 and 8 months	1941	65 and 4 months
65 and 10 months	1942	65 and 6 months
66	1943	65 and 8 months
66	1944	65 and 10 months
66	1945	66
66	1946	66
66	1947	66
66	1948	66
66	1949	66
66	1950	66
66	1951	66
66	1952	66
66	1953	66
66	1954	66
66 and 2 months	1955	66
66 and 4 months	1956	66
66 and 6 months	1957	66 and 2 months
66 and 8 months	1958	66 and 4 months
66 and 10 months	1959	66 and 6 months
67	1960	66 and 8 months
67	1961	66 and 10 months
67	1962 and after	67

Note: If you were born on January 1, refer to the year prior to the year of your birth.

Early Retirement

You can claim retirement benefits as early as the first **full** month that you are age 62 if you are fully insured (page 30). You will have a smaller monthly benefit though for the rest of your life, than if you wait until the Normal Retirement Age. It will be smaller for two reasons. First, you will probably have lower average earnings because you won't have the earnings of later years. Second, you will receive more monthly benefit checks because they will begin sooner. Accordingly, the benefit is reduced. This way, the total benefits you receive will have approximately the same value if you live to an "average" age.

How much your benefit will be reduced for early retirement depends on your age when the benefits begin. On the following page are some reduced amounts for certain ages and PIAs for people **born before 1938.** (The reductions are somewhat larger for people born after 1937, as discussed later.)

Examples of Your Reduced Benefits at Early Retirement

If You Retire at Age	You Will Receive This Percent of Your PIA	You Will Receive This Benefit if Your PIA Is:		
		$600	**$900**	**$1,200**
65	100	$600	$900	$1,200
64½	96⅔	580	870	1,160
64	93⅓	560	840	1,120
63½	90	540	810	1,080
63	86⅔	520	780	1,040
62½	83⅓	500	750	1,000
62	80	480	720	960

You may retire at ages between the ones shown. The reduction factor applied to the Primary Insurance Amount is $5/9$ of 1% for each of the first 36 months that commencement is prior to the Normal Retirement Age, plus $5/12$ of 1% for each such month in excess of 36. These reduction factors are for workers only.

For spouse's benefits, start with an amount equal to 50% of the worker's PIA. Then apply a reduction factor of $25/36$ of 1% for each of the first 36 months that commencement is prior to the spouse's Normal Retirement Age, plus $5/12$ of 1% for each such month in excess of 36 (see tables on page 51). A spouse's reduction is slightly larger than that of the worker because of a contingent benefit for which there is a cost — that is, on the death of the worker, the reduction no longer applies. Then, the spouse will be paid a much larger benefit — generally, an amount equal to the worker's benefit (pages 90-91).

Example of Spouse's Reduced Benefits at Early Retirement

Age Benefits Begin	Percentage of Worker's PIA Received	You Will Receive This Benefit if Worker's PIA Is:		
		$600	$900	$1,200
65	50	$300	$450	$600
64½	47.92	288	431	575
64	45.83	275	412	549
63½	43.75	263	394	525
63	41.67	250	375	500
62½	39.59	238	356	475
62	37.50	225	338	450

For a surviving spouse's benefit, the reduction factor applied to the Primary Insurance Amount of the deceased worker when the Normal Retirement Age is 65 is $^{19}/_{40}$ of 1% for each month that commencement is prior to the surviving spouse's Normal Retirement Age — to a maximum reduction of 28.5%. (The Normal Retirement Age is slightly different from that for workers and spouses — for example, age 67 for those born in 1962, or later (as compared with age 67 being the applicable age for workers and spouses born in 1960, or later). If the Normal Retirement Age is greater than 65, the benefit will be reduced by 28.5% prorated for the number of months that commencement of payment precedes the Normal Retirement Age as compared with the number of months between age 60 and the Normal Retirement Age. For example, if the Normal Retirement Age is 67, and the age when benefits are claimed is 63½, then benefits precede the Normal Retirement Age by 42 months (3½ years). This is one-half of the 84-month (7-year) period between age 60 and 67. Accordingly, the reduction is one-half of the 28.5% or 14.25%.

Reduction Factors for Early Retirement at Ages 62 and 65 for Workers and Spouses, Based on Year of Birth

(Factors for spouses apply to 50% of the worker's PIA)

First claiming benefits at age 62:

Year of Birth	Reduction Factor	
	Retired Worker	Spouse
1937 or before	20.00%	25.00%
1938	20.83	25.83
1939	21.67	26.67
1940	22.50	27.50
1941	23.33	28.33
1942	24.17	29.17
1943-54	25.00	30.00
1955	25.83	30.83
1956	26.67	31.67
1957	27.50	32.50
1958	28.33	33.33
1959	29.17	34.17
1960 or after	30.00	35.00

First claiming benefits at age 65:

Year of Birth	Reduction Factor	
	Retired Worker	Spouse
1937 or before	NONE	NONE
1938	1.11%	1.39
1939	2.22	2.78
1940	3.33	4.17
1941	4.44	5.56
1942	5.56	6.94
1943-54	6.67	8.33
1955	7.78	9.72
1956	8.89	11.11
1957	10.00	12.50
1958	11.11	13.89
1959	12.22	15.28
1960 or after	13.33	16.67

Reductions for Early Retirement Are Permanent

If your benefit is reduced because you started it before the Normal Retirement Age, the reduction is **permanent.** Your benefit does not increase to the full PIA when you reach Normal Retirement Age. However, if your benefit is reduced for any month that you have more **earnings** than Social Security allows (pages 60-64), this reduction will be adjusted at the Normal Retirement Age. Then, your benefit will be refigured so that the permanent reduction is no longer based on any months that your benefit was suspended, in whole or in part, because of your earnings.

Begin Social Security at 62?

One of the most commonly asked Social Security questions is whether retirement benefits should be started at age 62, or whether one should wait until later. People generally expect an easy "yes" or "no" answer, but unfortunately the question is not that simple. It depends on individual circumstances.

Beginning Social Security retirement benefits at the earliest permissible age of 62 as compared to the normal retirement age of 65 is intended to be an "actuarial equivalent." This means that workers, on average, come out the same financially under either alternative. However, actuarial equivalents depend on the current real rate of return on invested money (i.e., after allowing for price inflation) and also on the sex and health of the individual. Consequently, the 20% reduction of benefits at age 62 is only a form of "rough justice."

The mathematics of each case and the rate of return on invested money are important considerations. Equally important, however, are factors such as the need for the income at age 62, whether much work will be performed after age 62, the sex of the individual, whether the benefit is for a worker or spouse, the condition of health, and the expected longevity.

If one is no longer employed at age 62, and the income is essential, commencing benefits then is the right decision. If significant earnings after age 62 are expected, then deferring the commencement of benefits may be desirable rather than getting into the complications of the Social Security earnings limitation. For example, if one started benefits at age 62, went back to work six months later for one year, until age 65 he or she would still be charged the reduction factor for three years (20%) even though collecting "early" benefits for only two years.

With the growing popularity of defined contribution retirement plans (e.g., 401(k) thrift plans), retirement at age 62 might qualify one for a large lump-sum distribution. This may eliminate the cash-flow need to commence Social Security benefits early. On the other hand, deferring receipt of the distribution, or rolling it over into an Individual Retirement Account (IRA), may achieve additional tax deferred investment growth. Also, only part of the Social Security benefits are subject to income taxes, and for lower-income persons none is taxable.

Since women at age 65 have a life expectancy of about four years greater than men, a woman in good health (and not impoverished) can often "beat the odds" by deferring Social Security benefits based on her own work record until age 65.

With respect to spouse benefits, however, generally a woman should start the benefit at age 62 (if eligible), because in the event of her husband's death, she would be entitled to his larger benefit amount with no cost for having taken her spousal benefit early. Of course, "early" benefits for a wife often are a combination of her own earned benefits and those based on her husband's work — provided he has started his benefits. In this case, the portion based on her own work, would be reduced permanently.

Potential benefits for a surviving spouse require other facts to be considered. For example, if a husband commenced reduced benefits before the Normal Retirement Age (NRA) of 65, the "cost" will be higher if he leaves a widow with no significant work record of her own. At her NRA, she would **not** collect his full Primary Insurance Amount (PIA) but rather his reduced benefit (but not less than 82.5% of his PIA). On the other hand, at age 60, she can commence an actuarially reduced widow's benefits of 71.5% of her husband's PIA with no additional cost for her deceased husband having started his benefit early. Again, health conditions must be considered before making a judgment and also the difference in ages as between the spouses.

The health and family longevity factors are important. If the insured worker lives beyond the "normal" life expectancy, then receiving the full benefit (primary insurance amount) at age 65 is obviously advantageous.

For those looking for a purely analytical answer to their question, the mathematics is easy for an actuary, but not so simple for ordinary citizens. If a retired worker at age 62 invested all Social Security payments at a "real" rate of interest of $2\frac{1}{2}\%$, at age 80 he or she would have accumulated about the same amount of money as if commencement of benefits had been deferred to age 65 and the larger payments had been invested at the same rate of interest. Age 80 would be the life expectancy of a man at age 65. Taking a slightly different approach, at various assumed interest rates (e.g., 4%, 5%, and 6%), calculations could be made to determine how long one would have to live for the accumulated sums to be equal.

The fact that Social Security payments are now subject to income taxes in many cases is an added complication. While many pay nothing at all, some pay income tax on 50% of their benefits, some on 85%, and some at a combination of these rates. State laws vary.

Calculations can be made in individual cases but never with absolute certainty. Rates of return are not always guaranteed, longevity is never certain, and changes in the law may occur.

In general, eligible spouses should commence their benefit at age 62, female workers should generally defer theirs until 65, and for male workers, it's a "toss-up." The need for the money, condition of health and expected longevity are the critical factors.

Late Retirement

If you wait until after your Normal Retirement Age to claim your Social Security benefit, you will earn Delayed Retirement Credits (DRCs). Your benefit will be increased by the percentage factor shown below (prorated for months). This will also occur with respect to months when you completely lose benefits because of the earnings limitation (see pages 60-64). For birth years beginning in 1925, the annual percentage increase rises ½% each two years until it reaches 8%. The following table illustrates this important provision:

Year of Birth	Increase for Each Year That Benefits Are Delayed Beyond the Normal Retirement Age
1917-24	3.0%
1925-26	3.5%
1927-28	4.0%
1929-30	4.5%
1931-32	5.0%
1933-34	5.5%
1935-36	6.0%
1937-38	6.5%
1939-40	7.0%
1941-42	7.5%
1943 or later	8.0%

The benefit increase is prorated for partial years. For example, if you were born in 1935, the percentage increase is 6% per year or $\frac{1}{2}$% for each month of delayed retirement.

When the increase becomes 8%, this will be an "actuarial equivalent," which simply means that, for persons who live to an average life expectancy, the value of the benefit at the Normal Retirement Age will be the same as the value of the benefit if claimed at a later age. One effect of this will be to greatly reduce the importance of the Social Security earnings limitation (pages 60-64), because what you don't get "today" will be paid "tomorrow." The larger benefit may be needed when you are fully retired and without income from work; also, the benefit may be less likely to be fully or partially subjected to income taxes.

Earnings after the Normal Retirement Age may increase your AIME and, thus, your PIA. Any increase in your PIA will increase your benefits and those of family members who receive benefits based on your earnings. The percentage increase for delayed retirement, however, affects only the benefits paid to workers, and surviving spouses, and does not increase the current benefits of other family members.

Family Benefits

When you retire and become entitled to Social Security benefits, other members of your family may also become entitled to benefits based on your earnings record. Their benefits are figured as a percentage of your PIA (not necessarily your **benefit**) but are subject to the Maximum Family Benefit. Such maximum reduces all benefits except the worker's benefit. After the application of such maximum, your **retirement** benefit will be lower than your PIA if it begins before the Normal Retirement Age, and it will be larger than your PIA if you retire later. The following table shows the percentage of your PIA payable to your family members when you retire:

Who Receives Benefits When You Retire

Benefits Paid To	Percent of Your PIA Payable
Spouse, age 65*	50%
Spouse, age 62	37.5%**
Spouse, any age, with eligible child who is under age 16 or disabled	50%
Each eligible child	50%

* When the Normal Retirement Age for workers rises, this age will rise, too.

** Gradually reduced starting in the year 2000 (pages 51 and 153).

You must apply for benefits before your family members can become entitled to benefits (except as noted below for divorced spouses). The benefits payable to your family members are **in addition** to your own benefit. Let's look at the family members and the qualifications which they must meet:

Spouse

A spouse who first becomes entitled to Social Security at the Normal Retirement Age (NRA), will receive a benefit equal to 50% of your PIA. At age 62, your spouse can receive permanently reduced benefits, currently 37½% of your PIA (pages 49 and 153). You must begin your benefit before your spouse can collect a benefit on your work record.

If your spouse is also insured for a retirement benefit, then Social Security will pay that benefit first. The amount of the spouse benefit will be **limited** to the excess (if any) by which 50% of your PIA exceeds his or her own PIA. This excess is reduced if the spouse's benefit starts before the NRA. This spouse's benefit is then added to his or her own retirement benefit. This is done automatically by Social Security and is not a matter of choice.

A **spouse who is caring for your eligible child** is entitled to 50% of your PIA. The eligible child must be under age 16 (or any age, if disabled before age 22). In this case, no reduction is made because of the spouse's age. To qualify for benefits, your spouse must have been married to you for at least one year or must be the parent of your child.

Your **unmarried divorced spouse** may be entitled to benefits starting at age 62 if married to you for at least 10 years. This benefit is not payable if the divorced spouse is remarried, unless the marriage is to a person receiving benefits as a widow, widower, parent, or disabled child. These benefits are subject to the same reductions as spouse's benefits if they start before the Normal Retirement Age. A divorced spouse can receive benefits if you are at least age 62 (whether retired or not) or are receiving Social Security disability benefits. If you are 62 but not retired, then the divorce must have been at least two years ago before the divorced spouse can receive benefits unless you were entitled to benefits before the divorce.

Eligible Child

The definition of **child** includes your natural child, adopted child, stepchild, and dependent grandchild (if their parents are deceased or disabled). An eligible child must be unmarried and:

- under age 18; or
- age 18, if in high school; or
- any age, if disabled before age 22.

Each child is entitled to 50% of the parent's PIA — based on the PIA of either parent, whichever is greater, but not both.

Maximum Family Benefit

The total amount of benefits that all members of one family may receive based on the earnings record of one worker is limited to an amount that varies with the PIA. The table on pages 84 and 85 shows this **Maximum Family Benefit** for various AIMEs and PIAs for persons who reach age 62 in 1996 or who become disabled or die before age 62 in 1996. (The rule for calculating the maximum is on page 152.) The maximum is higher for retirement and survivor cases than for disability cases. The maximum applies before any reduction for early retirement or any increase for late retirement.

If the sum of the individual benefits based on your earnings record is more than the maximum, the benefits of the family members will be reduced proportionately to bring the total within the limit. Your worker's benefit will not be reduced. An example on pages 98-100 shows how this applies to survivor benefits.

The amount payable to a divorced spouse of a worker, whether or not the latter is alive, is not included in figuring the MFB, with one exception: the benefit of a surviving divorced spouse qualifying only on the basis of caring for a child of the worker **is** included in figuring the maximum.

Earnings Limitation for Employees (Retirement Test)

If you continue to work for an employer after your Social Security benefits start, your benefits may be reduced due to the Earnings Limitation, which is sometimes called the Retirement Test. It applies until you reach age 70.

Beginning with the year that your benefits start, you can earn up to a certain amount in each year without affecting your benefits in any way. But if you earn **more** than the Earnings Limitation, Social Security will reduce your benefits and your family members' benefits based on your work record. If a family member earns more than the Earnings Limitation, only that person's benefit is reduced.

In 1996, the Earnings Limitation for a beneficiary who is age 65-69 is $11,520. For beneficiaries under age 65 it is $8,280. These amounts increase every year, based on changes in the average earnings of all employees in the country.

If you are under age 65, benefits are reduced by $1 for every $2 you earn over the Earnings Limitation during the year. If you are 65-69, the reduction is $1 for every $3 you earn over the limitation. For example, let's assume that you are age 65 and start receiving Social Security retirement benefits in 1996. If you earn $41,520, this would be $30,000 over the permissible amount of $11,520. The loss in benefits would be $10,000 ($30,000 ÷ 3).

In the first year that there is a month in which you are both entitled to benefits and do not earn more than $1/12$ of the annual Earnings Limit, a monthly test is used **if it gives you better results** than the annual test just described. During that year, beginning with your month of entitlement, you can receive your benefit for any month that you do not earn more than $1/12$ of the Earnings Limitation. If you earn more than $1/12$ of the annual limit, benefits are not payable for that month unless they are payable under the regular annual test.

In some cases, you might continue working and also apply for retirement benefits, especially if family members are eligible for benefits on your earnings record. The benefits will be reduced because of the excess earnings, but this may be better than no benefits at all. Each case must be studied carefully to see whether the earnings after taxes are worth the reduction in benefits. Remember, too, that Social Security benefits are often tax free, while earnings are subject to federal, state, and local income taxes, as well as Social Security and Medicare taxes.

In the calendar year in which you plan to retire, you might consider applying for benefits in January, even if you have not stopped working yet (pages 32-34). If your total earnings for the calendar year are not more than the Earnings Limitation, you will get benefits for all months in that year after you are entitled to benefits (and, if over age 65, for some earlier months).

Earnings Limitation for Self-Employed

If you are self-employed, you also are subject to the Earnings Limitation until age 70. The annual limitation is the same as for employees. Under a special **alternative** test for the first year that you receive benefits and have, at the same time, a month when you do not perform substantial services in self-employment, your work is examined to determine such months. Then, benefits are paid for those months. In general, less than 15 hours of services in a month is not considered substantial; more than 45 hours of services in a month is considered substantial. Between those guidelines, your services are considered substantial if you are in a highly skilled occupation.

For the annual Earnings Limitation, the profits and losses of all your businesses are added together to determine the earnings for the year. If the total profit was over the Earnings Limitation, your Social Security benefits will be reduced, even if some of the businesses lost money.

Earnings from self-employment received after retirement are generally counted when you receive them, rather than when earned. However, earnings from work performed before the month of entitlement to retirement benefits do not count towards the Earnings Limitation (except that income received in the year of retirement counts for the annual limitation).

If you are self-employed and also employed by others, you must combine your salary and wages and your net income or loss from self-employment to see whether your earnings exceed the Earnings Limitation.

Income for Earnings Limitation

Certain types of income are **not** counted as earnings in applying the Earnings Limitation. Some of these are:

- pensions and retirement pay;
- 401(k) plan and IRA withdrawals;
- employee contributions pursuant to a salary reduction under a Section 125 cafeteria plan to fund a qualified benefit;
- payments from certain tax-exempt trust funds such as profit sharing, bond purchase, or annuity plans;
- severance payments made on account of retirement;
- dividends and interest from investments, unless you are in the brokerage business, and capital gains;
- rental income unless you are in the real estate business;
- non-cash payments for domestic service;
- tips not in cash or amounting to less than $20 in a month;
- sick pay if paid more than 6 months after the month last worked;
- workers' compensation and unemployment insurance benefits;
- reimbursement for travel or moving expenses to the extent they are not counted as income by Internal Revenue Service;
- damages, fees, interest, or penalties received in a court judgment, except *that back pay recovered must be counted as wages or salary;
- contest or lottery winnings; and
- vacation or bonus pay earned in a prior year.

Even if the Earnings Limitation causes a loss of the entire benefit for a period of time, Medicare coverage continues if you otherwise qualify.

You may receive some benefits retroactively for as many as six months but not for any month prior to your Normal Retirement Age. (For disability benefits, the retroactive period can be as much as 12 months.) This could happen if you were eligible for benefits but did not apply on time.

Because some payments made after retirement are subject to payroll taxes (pages 19-20), the Social Security Administration may erroneously believe that you are working and subject to the Earnings Limitation even if you have retired. The most common situations that can cause problems involve payments for accrued vacation pay, bonuses, and nonqualified deferred compensation arrangements. In such cases, you may need your former employer to document the types of payment that were made and whether they represented compensation for current services. Generally, payments for **past** services will not cause benefit reductions under the Earnings Limitation. Some large employers have arranged to tell the Social Security Administration automatically about such payments to prevent the standard inquiries from being sent to their retirees.

Annual Earnings Report Process

Social Security beneficiaries who earn over the allowable limit (under the rules of the annual earnings test — see pages 60-64) are required to file an Annual Report of Earnings with the Social Security Administration.

The deadline for filing this report is April 15 each year. Even though the deadline is the same as for filing your income tax return, it is a separate report. Your income tax return is filed with the Internal Revenue Service; your Annual Report of Earnings is filed with the Social Security Administration. Filing an income tax return DOES NOT satisfy the requirement of filing an Annual Report of Earnings with Social Security.

Social Security attempts to send the appropriate form to each affected beneficiary. If you do not receive this form in January, call Social Security at **800-772-1213.**

You can either complete the form and mail it to Social Security, or in most cases, provide the necessary information over the telephone.

The Annual Report of Earnings has two purposes. First, it is used to compare your actual earnings for the prior year with what you had estimated your earnings to be. This will enable Social Security to verify if you were paid the correct amount of benefits. If your actual earnings were less than what you had estimated, then Social Security may owe you additional benefits. If your actual earnings were more than you had estimated, then you may have been overpaid.

The second purpose of the Annual Report of Earnings is to get an estimate of your expected earnings for the current year. Social Security will use this information to determine what benefits you are due for the current year.

It is important to notify Social Security as soon as possible if there is a change in your estimated earnings. They will make any necessary adjustments in your benefits as new information is received. This can usually be done by telephone.

The Annual Report of Earnings process is usually simple for employees. It can be more complicated for those who own or control a business. Social Security may ask more detailed questions as circumstances warrant. Social Security recognizes that such persons sometimes have opportunity to disguise their actual earnings in attempts to circumvent the rules of the annual earnings test.

Reduction of Benefits Because of Other Pensions

The "Windfall" Elimination Provision

A provision of Social Security law, called the **windfall elimination,** modifies the method of computing the retirement or disability (but not survivor) PIA, resulting in lower benefit amounts. This applies to many people receiving pensions based on their own earnings from employment **not covered** by Social Security. This includes some government pensions, as well as pensions from foreign employment.

The purpose of the windfall elimination provision was to close a loophole that enabled people who worked in both covered and noncovered employment to receive the unintended advantage of the weighted Social Security PIA formula. The PIA formula is weighted in favor of the career low-level earner because such a person is more dependent on Social Security for retirement income needs than higher-income people. Such persons who work in both covered and noncovered employment appear to be low earners when only their covered earnings are considered, and thus they would receive large benefits in relation to such earnings if it were not for this provision.

It does not apply to:

- persons reaching age 62 before 1986;
- persons **eligible** for such pensions before 1986;
- disabled-worker beneficiaries disabled before 1986;
- persons with at least 30 years of substantial Social Security coverage (defined as follows);
- federal employees who were mandatorily covered by Social Security on January 1, 1984; and
- persons employed on January 1, 1984, by nonprofit organizations that were not covered by Social Security at any time before 1984.

The special computation method substitutes a lower factor for the 90% ordinarily applied to the first interval of the PIA formula (page 151). Except as noted below, the factor that is substituted is 80% for workers born in 1924; 70% for workers born in 1925; 60% for workers born in 1926; 50% for workers born in 1927; and 40% for workers born in 1928 and later.

For workers with at least 21 years of substantial Social Security covered earnings, a larger factor may be applicable, as follows:

Years of Work	Special Factor	Years of Work	Special Factor
30	90%	24	60%
29	85	23	55
28	80	22	50
27	75	21	45
26	70	20 or fewer	40
25	65		

Substantial earnings for each year are:

Year	Substantial Earnings	Year	Substantial Earnings
1937-50	$ 900	1981	$ 5,550
1951-54	900	1982	6,075
1955-58	1,050	1983	6,675
1959-65	1,200	1984	7,050
1966-67	1,650	1985	7,425
1968-71	1,950	1986	7,875
1972	2,250	1987	8,175
1973	2,700	1988	8,400
1974	3,300	1989	8,925
1975	3,525	1990	9,525
1976	3,825	1991	9,900
1977	4,125	1992	10,350
1978	4,425	1993	10,725
1979	4,725	1994	11,250
1980	5,100	1995	11,325
		1996	11,625

*Total credited earnings from 1937-50 are divided by $900 to get the number of years of coverage (maximum of 14 years).

The windfall elimination provision only modifies the PIA computation. Unlike the government-pension offset (discussed next), it cannot reduce the computed benefit to zero. Also, it does not apply to computing the PIA for survivor benefits.

Government Pension Offset (Spouses)

If **you** worked for federal, state, or local government and were **not covered by Social Security** when your employment ended, two-thirds of your pension benefits from that employment will be offset against any Social Security benefit for which you are eligible as a **spouse, widow,** or **widower.** You can receive only the amount of the Social Security benefit that exceeds two-thirds of your government pension. This frequently eliminates Social Security benefits altogether. This reduction rule does not apply to:

- persons entitled to Social Security benefits before December 1977;

- women, and men who were dependent on their wives, who received, or were eligible to receive, government pensions any time during December 1977 through November 1982; and

- persons eligible to receive government pensions during December 1982 through June 1983 who were dependent on their spouses.

This provision of the law is called the **government pension offset.** It is important to understand that this provision only applies to Social Security benefits that you receive as a dependent or survivor, not to benefits you earned as a worker. This offset also does not affect Medicare eligibility.

Example: Doris was a school teacher for 25 years and was never covered by Social Security. Her husband's Primary Insurance Amount is $1,000 a month. At age 65 or older, she is eligible to receive an amount equal to 50% of $1,000, or $500 a month. But her teacher's pension is $900, and two-thirds of this is $600, which exceeds the $500 amount. Thus she cannot receive a Social Security benefit on her husband's work record. If her teacher's pension were $600, two-thirds (or $400) would be offset against her $500 wife's benefit under Social Security, and she could collect $100 a month.

Many retired government employees affected by the government pension offset consider that they are being singled out for unfair treatment. In fact, the purpose of the law is to treat them similarly to other retirees who worked in Social Security covered employment. The amount of any dependent or survivor benefit payable under Social Security is offset by the amount of any Social Security retirement or disability benefit that a person receives based on his or her own earnings. For instance, in the example described, if Doris had earned a PIA of $500 or more on her own Social Security work record, she could not collect a benefit based on her husband's work record.

The government pension offset can reduce the Social Security spouse or survivor benefit to zero, but not always. Even if a spouse benefit is reduced to zero, this does not necessarily mean that, later, a higher survivor benefit would also be reduced to zero. Suppose, for instance, that Doris' husband dies. She would be eligible to receive his PIA of $1,000 a month, minus an amount equal to two-thirds of her teacher's pension.

It is important to apply for benefits and let Social Security make a formal determination. Don't just assume that you aren't eligible. Also, if your benefit is reduced to zero, you can still qualify for Medicare Part A.

Minimum Retirement Benefits

Special-Minimum Benefit (Long Service at Low Earnings)

Workers who have many years of work under Social Security, but at low earnings, may qualify for a **special-minimum benefit.** The amount of the PIA for this benefit depends on the number of years of "significant" Social Security coverage. Here's how that PIA is figured:

For 1937-50, divide your total earnings by $900 to obtain your years of coverage (maximum 14). For 1951-78, you were credited for each year that you earned at least 25% of the Maximum Taxable Earnings. For 1979-90, you are credited for each year that you earned about 19% of the Maximum Taxable Earnings. After 1990, it is about 11%. For 1996, you are credited with a year of coverage if you earn at least $6,975.

For December 1995 through November 1996, the special-minimum benefit is *approximately* $26.65 per month for each year of coverage **over 10 years — up to 30 years.** Thus, for 11 years of coverage, the special-minimum PIA is $26.40, while for 30 or more years of coverage, it is $532.90.

For those retiring before the Normal Retirement Age, the benefit is reduced by applying reduction factors to the PIA (see pages 48-51). However, for those delaying retirement after such age, no increases are given (see page 55 for such increases for the regular method of computing the PIA).

The special-minimum benefit is paid only if it is higher than the benefit calculated under the regular rules, described previously, and this is seldom the case. The Social Security Administration automatically calculates your benefit, using both methods, and pays whichever is higher.

Example — Retirement Benefits

Married Couple:	Joe	Marilyn
Born	1935	1934
Age 62 in	1997	1996
PIA	$1,000	$400*

* **Note:** Marilyn was not employed when her children were young, and stopped her employment several years before reaching age 62.

At age 62, Marilyn can receive a benefit on her own earnings record. She doesn't have to wait for Joe to retire. Her PIA is $400. Because she is starting her benefit before age 65, it is reduced by $5/9$ of 1% for each month — or a reduction of 20% for 36 months. This reduces her monthly benefit to $320 at age 62. Marilyn could continue to receive this amount, plus cost-of-living increases (applicable also in all of the following cases), for the rest of her life. However, when Joe retires, she will receive a larger monthly benefit based partly on **his** earnings record.

If Joe retires next year at age 62, his PIA will be $1,000. This must be reduced in the same way that Marilyn's was (20% for the three years before age 65), resulting in a monthly benefit of $800. If Joe remains retired, he'll receive this amount for the rest of his life.

If Joe claims his benefit at age 62 but continues to work and earns more than the Earnings Limitation, his benefit would be further reduced (pages 60-61), as would Marilyn's spouse benefit. Her benefit based on **her** work record, however, is not affected by Joe's earnings.

When Joe reaches age 65, his benefit and Marilyn's spouse benefit will be increased to recognize any months in which benefits were withheld or reduced because of his work. If he continues to work after age 65, he will receive delayed retirement credits for months when benefits are withheld completely (page 55). Also, the additional years of earnings after age 62 would probably raise his PIA above $1,000.

Marilyn can collect benefits based on Joe's work record **whenever** he retires. If her wife's benefit begins at age 65, she may receive an amount up to 50% of Joe's PIA — or $500. If Marilyn had no work history under Social Security, she would receive this amount each month. However, Marilyn has earned a PIA of $400, which must be subtracted from the $500, resulting in a spouse's benefit of $100.

If she claims this benefit before age 65, it will be reduced by $^{25}/_{36}$ of 1% for each month. This reduction is different from the one used for her own PIA (page 50). At age 63, the reduction would be $16^2/_3$%, or about $17, resulting in a spouse's benefit of $83. Combined with her own benefit of $320 started at age 62, she would receive $403 a month while both she and Joe are alive.

If Joe and Marilyn both wait until age 65 to receive benefits, even though he stopped working at age 62, each would receive the full PIAs they had earned — $1,000 for Joe and $400 for Marilyn. In addition, Marilyn would receive a spouse's benefit of $100, which brings her total payments to $500 — an amount equal to 50% of Joe's PIA.

If Joe had had the lower earnings record, and Marilyn had had the higher earnings record, the total benefit payments would be the same as in the example described.

5

Disability Benefits

If you have worked long enough under Social Security and become severely disabled more than six months before attaining your Normal Retirement Age (NRA), you can receive a monthly disability benefit which is equal to what your PIA was at the time that the disability occurred. The benefit is not reduced because it starts before the NRA, currently 65. However, if you become disabled after age 62 and have already received a reduced retirement benefit, your disability benefit will be reduced to take into account the number of months you received the retirement benefit.

Easy-Reference Table

The table on the next page shows the approximate benefits for you and your family if you become disabled in 1996. The figures assume that you have worked steadily and received average pay raises throughout your working career. By following the steps described on pages 78-81, you can make a more accurate calculation.

Like other Social Security benefits, disability benefits are increased each year to reflect changes in the cost of living.

A Maximum Family Benefit (page 59) applies, and this can be determined from the table on pages 84-85 by finding your PIA in column 2 and looking across to the last column. In all the examples shown below, the maximum is 150% of the benefit shown for you (which is the PIA).

Monthly Benefits at Disability

Your Age in 1996	Who Receives Benefits	Your Present Annual Earnings				
		$15,000	$24,000	$36,000	$48,000	$62,700 and Up
64*	You	$636	$863	$1,125	$1,205	$1,275
	Child (or children & spouse)	318	431	562	602	637
60	You	624	846	1,106	1,189	1,262
	Child (or children & spouse)	312	423	553	594	631
55	You	624	846	1,113	1,212	1,297
	Child (or children & spouse)	312	423	556	606	648
50	You	624	846	1,118	1,238	1,342
	Child (or children & spouse)	312	423	559	619	671
45	You	624	847	1,118	1,252	1,377
	Child (or children & spouse)	312	423	559	626	688
40	You	624	847	1,119	1,258	1,411
	Child (or children & spouse)	312	423	559	629	705
35	You	624	848	1,119	1,258	1,425
	Child (or children & spouse)	312	424	559	629	712
30	You	625	848	1,120	1,259	1,435
	Child (or children & spouse)	312	424	560	629	717

* Disability benefits are not paid to persons 65 or over.

Qualifications for Disability Benefits

Disability means that you are so severely impaired, mentally or physically, that you cannot perform any substantial gainful work. The impairment must be expected to last at least 12 months or to result in earlier death. This determination must be based on medical evidence and is ordinarily made by a government agency in your state.

To qualify for disability benefits, you must have earned a minimum number of credits of Social Security coverage (as defined on page 30). In addition, you must have earned some of these credits in recent years.

The following table summarizes the requirements for anyone becoming disabled in 1996. If you were born on January 1, refer to the year prior to the year of your birth.

Year of Birth	Credits Required To Qualify for Disability Benefits in 1996
1931-34	40, with 20 earned in last 10 years
1935	39, with 20 earned in last 10 years
1936	38, with 20 earned in last 10 years
1937	37, with 20 earned in last 10 years
1938	36, with 20 earned in last 10 years
1939	35, with 20 earned in last 10 years
1940	34, with 20 earned in last 10 years
1941	33, with 20 earned in last 10 years
1942	32, with 20 earned in last 10 years
1943	31, with 20 earned in last 10 years
1944	30, with 20 earned in last 10 years
1945	29, with 20 earned in last 10 years
1946	28, with 20 earned in last 10 years
1947	27, with 20 earned in last 10 years
1948	26, with 20 earned in last 10 years
1949	25, with 20 earned in last 10 years
1950	24, with 20 earned in last 10 years
1951	23, with 20 earned in last 10 years
1952	22, with 20 earned in last 10 years
1953	21, with 20 earned in last 10 years
1954-65*	20 earned in last 10 years
1966*	19 earned after age 21
1967*	17 earned after age 21
1968*	15 earned after age 21
1969*	13 earned after age 21
1970*	11 earned after age 21
1971*	9 earned after age 21
1972*	7 earned after age 21
After 1972	6 earned in last 3 years

*The figure shown is the maximum number of credits required. Depending on month of birth and month of disability, the number can be up to 3 fewer, with a minimum of 6 credits.

Waiting Period

Disability benefits begin after a waiting period of five full calendar months. To qualify for benefits, you must have been disabled throughout this period. For example, if you become disabled on March 15, you could not receive benefits for March or the next five months, April through August. The first benefit would be for September and would normally be paid on October 3. If you previously received disability benefits and the disability ended less than five years before the present disability began, you will not have a second waiting period.

Disability benefits can be paid retroactively for up to 12 months, not including the waiting period. If a disabled worker dies before filing a claim, the family can apply for the disability benefits within three months of the worker's death.

Family Benefits

If you become disabled, your family members can receive benefits under the same rules that would apply if you retired (page 57). The Maximum Family Benefit, including your benefit, is generally 150% of your PIA. This is lower than for retirement and survivor benefits (pages 59-60, 84-85 and 152).

The following table shows the percentage of your PIA payable to your family members if you qualify for disability benefits.

Benefits Paid To	Percent of Your PIA Payable
Spouse, age 65*	50%
Spouse, age 62	37.5%**
Spouse with child under 16 or disabled	50%
Each eligible child	50%

* When the Normal Retirement Age for workers rises, this age will rise, too.

** Gradually reduced starting in the year 2000 (pages 51 and 139).

Rehabilitation
When you apply for disability benefits, you may be referred to the appropriate state agency for rehabilitation services.

Workers' Compensation
The law provides for a possible reduction in disability benefits when you have been awarded workers' compensation or certain other disability benefits under federal, state, or local law. The total of all such disability benefits may not exceed 80% of your recent earnings before your disability began. Benefits from the Department of Veterans Affairs based on financial need and benefits based on government employment covered by Social Security do not cause any reduction.

Earnings Limitation
The usual earnings limitation (pages 60-64) does not apply to disabled beneficiaries. It does apply, however, to working spouses and children who receive benefits as the dependents of disabled beneficiaries.

Trial Work
If you are a disabled beneficiary, you are encouraged to go back to work, if you are able to. However, you must notify Social Security of all work attempts. Benefits can continue throughout a nine-month (not necessarily consecutive) trial work period, plus an additional three-month grace period. A month in which earnings exceed $200 generally counts as a month of trial work.

After completion of the trial work period, additional earnings are evaluated to determine if they are substantial. Earnings in excess of $500 a month generally constitute substantial gainful work. The threshold for blind beneficiaries is $960. After the three-month grace period, benefits are suspended if earnings are considered substantial. Benefits can be reinstated during a 36-month extended period of eligibility for any month that earnings do not exceed $500.

Medicare coverage can continue for at least 39 months after completion of the trial work period.

Anyone under 65 who continues to have a disabling impairment, and who has lost Medicare coverage after 36 months due to work, can purchase Parts A and B by paying the monthly premiums (pages 104 and 109).

How To Figure Your Disability Benefit Amount

Your disability benefit equals your PIA at the time that disability occurs. To figure your PIA, you need to know your earnings history, because your PIA is based on your Average Indexed Monthly Earnings (AIME). By following the steps below, you can figure your own AIME. This, in turn, will give you a good estimate of your PIA if you become disabled in 1996. The following instructions do not apply to persons born before 1934.

Here's how to figure your AIME:

(1)   In column C of the worksheet on page 81, enter your earnings for each year through 1995. **You can get past information from the Earnings and Benefit Estimate Statement** that you can receive from Social Security (page 176). If your earnings for any year were more than the Maximum Taxable Amount, use the Maximum Taxable Amount.

(2)   Multiply earnings for all years by the Index Factors in column D. The index factors make past earnings comparable to the level of earnings today. Enter the results of your multiplication in column E, Indexed Earnings.

(3)   Not all indexed earnings are used to figure your AIME. The table on the next page shows how many years of earnings to use if you become disabled in 1996. If you were born on January 1, refer to the year prior to the year of your birth. (The rule for determining how many years to use is on page 151.) If you are disabled after age 24 but before age 37, you may reduce the number of years shown by one for each year in which a child of yours (or of your spouse)

under age 3 lived in your home, and you were not employed (up to a maximum of 2 years if you are age 26-31 and of 1 year if you are age 25 or age 32-36).

Number of Years Used To Figure
Average Indexed Monthly Earnings

Year of Birth	Number of Years	Year of Birth	Number of Years
1931-34	35	1953	17
1935	34	1954	16
1936	33	1955	16
1937	32	1956	15
1938	31	1957	14
1939	30	1958	13
1940	29	1959	12
1941	28	1960	12
1942	27	1961	11
1943	26	1962	10
1944	25	1963	9
1945	24	1964	8
1946	23	1965	8
1947	22	1966	7
1948	21	1967	6
1949	20	1968	5
1950	20	1969	4
1951	19	1970	4
1952	18	1971	3
		After 1971	2

Enter the number of years you must use ...

(4) On the worksheet, put a check mark in column F, High Years, by the years of your highest indexed earnings in column E until you have checked the number of years you must use from (3).

(5) Add up all the indexed earnings in column E for the years you have checked in column F. ....$ _____

(6) Multiply the number of years in (3) by 12 to get months. ... _____

(7) Divide the total earnings shown in (5) by the months shown in (6) to get your AIME (drop cents). ....$ _____

Now, to figure your PIA:

(8) Look at the table on pages 84-85. Find your AIME from (7) as closely as possible in the first column of the table. The numbers on this line show your approximate PIA and the disability benefits based on it. For a more precise benefit determination, apply the 1996 benefit formula shown on page 151. The benefit amount is increased by the cost-of-living percentage effective for December each year and normally payable early in January. A different method of computing the PIA in connection with disability benefits (producing lower amounts) applies to people receiving a pension based on their earnings from noncovered employment — see page 66.

Worksheet for Figuring Your Indexed Earnings

A Calendar Year	B Maximum Taxable Amount	C Enter Your Taxable Earnings	×	D Index Factor	=	E Indexed Earnings	F High Years
1951	$ 3,600			8.48595			
1952	3,600			7.98889			
1953	3,600			7.56617			
1954	3,600			7.52733			
1955	4,200			7.19490			
1956	4,200			6.72455			
1957	4,200			6.52261			
1958	4,200			6.46566			
1959	4,800			6.16047			
1960	4,800			5.92783			
1961	4,800			5.81231			
1962	4,800			5.53515			
1963	4,800			5.40266			
1964	4,800			5.19053			
1965	4,800			5.09872			
1966	6,600			4.81000			
1967	6,600			4.55621			
1968	7,800			4.26320			
1969	7,800			4.03028			
1970	7,800			3.83974			
1971	7,800			3.65603			
1972	9,000			3.32972			
1973	10,800			3.13364			
1974	13,200			2.95782			
1975	14,100			2.75214			
1976	15,300			2.57450			
1977	16,500			2.42893			
1978	17,700			2.25023			
1979	22,900			2.06922			
1980	25,900			1.89824			
1981	29,700			1.72463			
1982	32,400			1.63464			
1983	35,700			1.55871			
1984	37,800			1.47217			
1985	39,600			1.41201			
1986	42,000			1.37131			
1987	43,800			1.28910			
1988	45,000			1.22859			
1989	48,000			1.18179			
1990	51,300			1.12962			
1991	53,400			1.08903			
1992	55,500			1.03567			
1993	57,600			1.02684			
1994	60,600			1.00000			
1995	61,200			1.00000			

Note: Index factors change each year based on change in U.S. average wage.

Example — Disability Benefits

Jim and His Family

Jim is disabled at age 44 in 1996. His PIA is $900. He has a wife, Donna, age 44; a son, Steve, age 12; and a son, Mike, age 8.

Jim's Qualifications for Disability Benefits

When Jim became disabled, he had earned 60 credits of Social Security coverage since he was 21, including 20 in the last 10 years. He had enough credits to be eligible for benefits.

He was disabled on January 15 and had to wait five full calendar months — February through June — until his benefit began. His first check, which was for July, came on August 3.

Jim is entitled to his PIA of $900, with no reduction because of his age, plus cost-of-living increases. Each of the three other members of Jim's family would be entitled to $450, which is an amount equal to 50% of Jim's PIA. This adds up to a total of $2,250, which is over the Maximum Family Benefit of $1,350. Jim can receive his full benefit of $900, but each family member receives $150.

Benefits Payable

Jim	$ 900
Donna	150
Steve	150
Mike	150
Total	$1,350

Jim, Two Years Later (1998)

Jim, still disabled, becomes eligible for Medicare in July 1998, even though he's far from 65 years old. Jim's family is not eligible for Medicare, however.

Six Years Later (2002)
Steve's benefit stops when he reaches age 18 and completes high school. Because the family benefit is still 150% of the PIA, the total remains the same. Jim receives $900; Donna receives $225; Mike receives $225.

Eight Years Later (2004)
Social Security reviews the case periodically to see if Jim, age 52, remains disabled. His disability continues.

Jim's youngest child, Mike, is 16. Donna's benefit stops because she is no longer caring for a child under age 16.

If Mike is still in high school, his benefit can continue until age 19; otherwise, it stops at age 18.

Jim and Donna, Age 62 in 2014
At 62, Donna is again eligible for benefits as Jim's wife. She is entitled to an amount equal to 50% of Jim's PIA when she is 66, which is the Normal Retirement Age for workers and spouses born in 1952. However, because she is receiving the benefit at 62, it is reduced by 30%, and she receives $315.

Jim continues to receive his PIA of $900 as a disability benefit. Their total income is $1,215.

Jim and Donna, Age 66 in 2018
Jim's disability benefit stops when he reaches Normal Retirement Age, but his retirement benefit begins automatically. It's the same amount — $900.

If Donna had waited until 66 to receive her benefit, she would have been entitled to the full 50% of Jim's PIA, or $450.

Their total retirement benefit would then have been:

$ 900	Jim's benefit
450	Donna's benefit
$1,350	Total retirement income

6 Table of Monthly Social Security Benefits with Respect to Persons Reaching Age 62, or Dying or Becoming Disabled Before Age 62, in 1996[1]

(If your exact AIME is not shown, your benefit will be between the benefits for the AIMEs just above and below your AIME.)

	Benefits for Workers and Their Families					Benefits for Survivors of Deceased Workers					
			Benefits for Family Members			Spouse[3] not Caring for Child					
			Spouse[3] Not Caring for Child		Child or Spouse[3] Caring for Child					Maximum Family Benefit for Retirement and Survivors[5]	Maximum Family Benefit for Disability
Average Indexed Monthly Earnings (AIME)	Age-65 Retirement Benefit or Disability Benefit[2]	Age-62 Retirement Benefit	Age 65	Age 62		Age 65[4]	Age 60 or Age 50-59 and Disabled	One Child	Spouse[3] and One Child, or Two Children		
	100% of PIA	80% of PIA	50% of PIA	37½% of PIA	50% of PIA	100% of PIA	71½% of PIA	75% of PIA	150% of PIA	150-188% of PIA	100-150% of PIA
$ 800	$ 509	$407	$254	$191	$254	$ 509	$364	$382	$ 764	$ 764	$ 680
900	541	433	270	203	270	541	387	406	812	812	765
1,000	573	458	286	215	286	573	409	430	860	877	850
1,100	605	484	302	227	302	605	432	454	908	964	908
1,200	637	509	318	239	318	637	455	478	956	1,051	956
1,300	669	535	334	251	334	669	478	502	1,004	1,138	1,004
1,400	701	561	350	263	350	701	501	526	1,052	1,225	1,052
1,500	733	586	366	275	366	733	524	550	1,100	1,312	1,100
1,600	765	612	382	287	382	765	547	574	1,148	1,399	1,148
1,700	797	637	398	299	398	797	570	598	1,196	1,486	1,196
1,800	829	663	414	311	414	829	593	622	1,244	1,541	1,244
1,900	861	689	430	323	430	861	615	646	1,292	1,584	1,292

2,000	893	714	446	335	446	893	638	670	1,340	1,627	1,340
2,100	925	740	462	347	462	925	661	694	1,388	1,670	1,388
2,200	957	765	478	359	478	957	684	718	1,436	1,713	1,436
2,300	989	791	494	371	494	989	707	742	1,484	1,756	1,484
2,500	1,053	842	526	395	526	1,053	753	790	1,580	1,842	1,580
2,700	1,106	885	553	414	553	1,106	791	829	1,658	1,935	1,659
2,900	1,136	909	568	426	568	1,136	812	852	1,704	1,987	1,704
3,100	1,166	933	583	437	583	1,166	833	874	1,748	2,040	1,749
3,300	1,196	957	598	448	598	1,196	855	897	1,794	2,092	1,794
3,500	1,226	981	613	459	613	1,226	876	919	1,838	2,145	1,839
3,657[6]	1,249	999	624	468	624	1,249	893	937	1,874	2,186	1,874

All numbers are rounded to the next lower whole dollar, in accordance with Social Security law. The Primary Insurance Amount (PIA) formula, the Maximum Family Benefit (MFB) formula, and the reduction factors for early retirement are shown on pages 151-153.

[1] For persons who were 62 before 1996, see Item (7) on page 151. **Benefits are increased annually for changes in the cost of living in and after the first year of eligibility (e.g., becoming age 62).**

[2] The disability benefit for a worker is the PIA, unless the worker was already receiving a benefit reduced for early retirement.

[3] Divorced spouses who qualify receive the same benefits as spouses. Benefits for divorced spouses are not ordinarily subject to the family maximum, however.

[4] A surviving spouse's benefit at age 65 is the PIA, unless the worker was receiving a benefit reduced for early retirement. In that case, the benefit will be the reduced amount that the worker was receiving, but not less than 82½% of the PIA.

[5] Any reduction for retirement before age 65 for workers, spouses, and surviving spouses is deducted.

[6] The maximum AIME for persons reaching age 62 in 1996 is generally $3,657, resulting in an age-62 benefit of $999 and an age-65 benefit of $1,249, assuming no earnings at ages 62-64. (For persons reaching age 65 in 1996, the maximum AIME is $3,402; a different table is used to obtain the monthly benefit amounts, and the maximum age-65 benefit is $1,248. See table on page 27.)

Note: Under some circumstances (generally, for younger, highly paid workers), persons who become disabled or die before age 62 can have higher AIMEs than $3,657. For example, at the extreme, a worker dying at age 24 or under in 1996 can have an AIME as high as $5,162 and a PIA of $1,475.

7

Survivor Benefits

The amount of the benefits payable to your survivors is based on your PIA on the date of your death.

Easy-Reference Table

The table on the next page shows the approximate monthly benefit amounts payable to your family members if you die in 1996. The figures are based on the assumption that you have worked steadily and received average pay raises throughout your working career. By following the steps described on pages 94-97, you can make a more accurate calculation.

Like other Social Security benefits, survivor benefits are increased each year to reflect changes in the cost of living.

Monthly Benefits if You Die in 1996

Your Age in 1996	Who Receives Benefits	Your Present Annual Earnings				
		$15,000	$24,000	$36,000	$48,000	$62,700 and Up
65	Spouse, age 65	$ 622	$ 845	$1,100	$1,179	$1,248
	Spouse, age 60	445	604	786	843	892
	Child; spouse caring for child	467	634	825	884	936
	Maximum family benefit	1,016	1,561	1,924	2,063	2,184
60	Spouse, age 65	624	846	1,106	1,189	1,262
	Spouse, age 60	446	605	790	850	902
	Child; spouse caring for child	468	634	829	892	946
	Maximum family benefit	1,015	1,564	1,934	2,080	2,207
55	Spouse, age 65	624	846	1,113	1,212	1,297
	Spouse, age 60	446	605	796	866	927
	Child; spouse caring for child	468	635	835	909	973
	Maximum family benefit	1,015	1,564	1,948	2,120	2,270
50	Spouse, age 65	624	846	1,118	1,238	1,342
	Spouse, age 60	446	605	799	885	959
	Child; spouse caring for child	468	635	839	928	1,006
	Maximum family benefit	1,016	1,564	1,956	2,166	2,348
45	Spouse, age 65	624	847	1,118	1,254	1,387
	Spouse, age 60	446	605	799	897	992
	Child; spouse caring for child	468	635	839	941	1,040
	Maximum family benefit	1,016	1,565	1,956	2,195	2,427
40	Spouse, age 65	624	847	1,119	1,258	1,420
	Spouse, age 60	446	606	800	899	1,015
	Child; spouse caring for child	468	635	839	943	1,065
	Maximum family benefit	1,016	1,566	1,957	2,201	2,484
35	Spouse, age 65	625	848	1,119	1,259	1,433
	Spouse, age 60	447	606	800	900	1,025
	Child; spouse caring for child	468	636	839	944	1,075
	Maximum family benefit	1,018	1,567	1,958	2,203	2,508
30	Spouse, age 65	628	853	1,123	1,264	1,455
	Spouse, age 60	449	610	803	903	1,040
	Child; spouse caring for child	471	640	842	948	1,091
	Maximum family benefit	1,027	1,573	1,964	2,210	2,545

Lump-Sum Death Benefit

When you die, whether still working or retired, a lump sum of $255 is payable to a surviving spouse who was living with you at the time of death. If you don't have a spouse living with you, then payment may be made to a spouse or children who are immediately eligible for monthly benefits based on your earnings record. Otherwise, the benefit is not payable.

Qualifications for Survivor Benefits

For your survivors to receive monthly benefits or the lump-sum death payment, you must be either:

- currently insured (provides eligibility for some benefits, but not all), or
- fully insured (provides eligibility for all benefits).

Currently Insured

To be currently insured, you need to have earned six credits during the 13 calendar quarters ending with the quarter in which you die.

If you are **currently insured,** the lump-sum death benefit is payable, and the following survivors qualify for monthly benefits:

- a spouse or divorced spouse caring for an eligible child who is under age 16 or disabled before age 22, and
- any eligible children under age 18; or age 18, if in high school; or disabled before age 22.

Fully Insured

The following table shows how many credits you need to be **fully insured.** To use the table, find your year of birth. Next to it is the number of credits you must have if you die in 1996. For example, if you were born in 1940, you need 34 credits to be fully insured. If you were born on January 1, refer to the year prior to the year of your birth. (The rule for determining the number of credits required is on page 151.)

Credits Required To Be Fully Insured if You Die in 1996

Year of Birth	Credits	Year of Birth	Credits
1926	37	1950	24
1927	38	1951	23
1928	39	1952	22
1929-34	40	1953	21
1935	39	1954	20
1936	38	1955	19
1937	37	1956	18
1938	36	1957	17
1939	35	1958	16
1940	34	1959	15
1941	33	1960	14
1942	32	1961	13
1943	31	1962	12
1944	30	1963	11
1945	29	1964	10
1946	28	1965	9
1947	27	1966	8
1948	26	1967	7
1949	25	After 1967	6

Family Benefits

Here are some examples of surviving family members who may receive benefits based on your PIA. The table also shows the percentage of your PIA ordinarily payable to each member.

Who Receives Benefits if You Die

Benefits Paid To	Percent of Your PIA Payable
Spouse, age 65*	100%
Spouse, age 62	82.9%**
Spouse, age 60	71.5%
Disabled spouse, age 50-59	71.5%
Spouse, under age 61 with eligible child who is under age 16 or disabled	75%
Each eligible child	75%

* When the Normal Retirement Age for workers rises (pages 47 and 139), this age will rise, too (but starting two years later); also, see the following discussion if you receive reduced retirement benefits.

** Slightly reduced, starting in 2002 (pages 51 and 153).

Eligibility

Your spouse qualifies for survivor benefits if:

- married to you for at least nine months before your death (if death is due to an accident or military duty, no length of marriage is required), or

- the parent of your child (natural or adopted).

Surviving Spouse, Age 60 or Over

If you die before you are entitled to retirement benefits, or after retiring at the Normal Retirement Age (NRA), the benefit is 100% of your PIA if your spouse has reached NRA. If your spouse is younger, a reduction applies (pages 50 and 153). However, if you retired before the NRA and had a reduced benefit, your spouse will receive the **smaller** of:

- 100% of your PIA, but reduced if your spouse is under the NRA or

- the reduced benefit that you were receiving (but in no case less than 82½% of your PIA).

If you retired after the NRA, your spouse will receive the same benefit (including the delayed retirement credit) that you had, but reduced if your spouse is under the NRA at the time of your death.

Your **divorced spouse** qualifies for a benefit if married to you for 10 years. The benefit is the same as that payable to a spouse.

If your surviving spouse or surviving divorced spouse remarries before age 60, benefits are not payable unless the subsequent marriage ends. Remarriage after attaining age 60 does not prevent or stop entitlement to benefits.

Disabled Surviving Spouse

Your **disabled spouse** age 50-59 who meets the definition of disability (see page 74) will qualify for benefits if the disability has lasted five full months. The benefit is 71½% of your PIA.

Your **disabled divorced spouse** qualifies in the same way as a disabled spouse if the marriage lasted at least 10 years.

Remarriage by your disabled surviving spouse or disabled surviving divorced spouse after age 50 and after the date he or she became disabled, does not prevent or stop entitlement to benefits.

Surviving Spouse Caring for Child

Your **spouse or divorced spouse caring for an eligible child** who is under age 16, or disabled before age 22, receives 75% of your PIA. The benefit stops when the youngest child reaches age 16, unless caring for an eligible child who was disabled before age 22. Your divorced spouse is not required to have been married to you for a specified length of time for this type of benefit. Remarriage terminates the benefit.

Eligible Child

An eligible child (page 59), qualifies for a benefit of 75% of the deceased parent's PIA. If both parents are dead, a child can qualify for benefits on the earnings record of either the mother or father, whichever gives the larger benefit. If the child gets married, the benefit usually terminates.

Dependent Parents

Your mother or father age 62 or over can qualify for survivor benefits if, at the time of your death, he or she was receiving at least one-half support from you. The benefit is 82½% of your PIA. However, if both parents are entitled to benefits, each receives 75%.

Maximum Family Benefit

The Maximum Family Benefit described on page 59 applies.

Non-Duplication of Benefits

A person eligible for more than one Social Security benefit for a particular month receives, in effect, the larger of the two benefits. For example, a widow of a deceased worker may receive a retirement benefit based on her own work record or a widow's benefit, but not both amounts.

Earnings Limitation

Anyone receiving survivor benefits (except on account of disability) is subject to the same Earnings Limitation as is applicable to those receiving retirement benefits and will lose benefits if earnings exceed the limit. This is especially applicable in the case of employed young widows with eligible children. If a family member earns more than the limitation, this does not reduce the benefits of the other family members, and in some cases will not even reduce the total family benefits. See pages 60-64 for a full explanation of this limitation.

Spouse Government Pension Offset

Surviving spouses who are entitled to a government pension based on employment not covered by Social Security may have their survivor benefit offset (page 68).

How To Figure Survivor Benefits

Survivor benefits are based on your PIA at the time of your death. To figure your PIA, you need to know your earnings history, because your PIA is based on your Average Indexed Monthly Earnings (AIME). By following the steps below, you can figure your own AIME. This, in turn, will give you a good estimate of your PIA if you die in 1996. The following instructions do not apply to persons born before 1934.

Here's how to figure your AIME:

(1) In column C of the worksheet on page 97, enter your earnings for each year, including 1996. **You can get past information from the Earnings and Benefit Estimate Statement** that you can receive from the Social Security Administration (page 176). If your earnings for any year were more than the Maximum Taxable Amount, use the Maximum Taxable Amount.

(2) Multiply your earnings for all years by the Index Factors in column D. The index factors make past earnings comparable to the level of earnings today. Enter the results of your multiplication in column E, Indexed Earnings.

(3) Not all indexed earnings are used to figure your AIME. The table on the next page shows how many years of earnings to use for death in 1996. If you were born on January 1, refer to the year prior to the year of your birth. (The rule for determining the number of years to use is on page 151.)

Number of Years Used To Figure
Average Indexed Monthly Earnings

Year of Birth	Number of Years	Year of Birth	Number of Years
1926	32	1950	19
1927	33	1951	18
1928	34	1952	17
1929-34	35	1953	16
1935	34	1954	15
1936	33	1955	14
1937	32	1956	13
1938	31	1957	12
1939	30	1958	11
1940	29	1959	10
1941	28	1960	9
1942	27	1961	8
1943	26	1962	7
1944	25	1963	6
1945	24	1964	5
1946	23	1965	4
1947	22	1966	3
1948	21	After 1966	2
1949	20		

Enter the number of years you must use ... _____

(4) On the worksheet, put a check mark in column F, High Years, by the years of your highest indexed earnings in column E until you have checked the number of years you must use from (3).

(5) Add up all the indexed earnings in column E for the years you have checked in column F. . . . $_____

(6) Multiply the number of years in (3) by 12 to get months. . . . _____

(7) Divide the total earnings shown in (5) by the months shown in (6) to get your AIME (drop cents). . . . $_____

Now, to figure your PIA:

(8) Look at the table on pages 84-85. Find your AIME from (7) as closely as possible in the first column of the table. The numbers on this line are your approximate PIA and the survivor benefits based on it. For a more precise benefit determination, apply the 1996 benefit formula shown on page 151. The benefit amount is increased by the cost-of-living percentage effective for December each year and normally payable early in January.

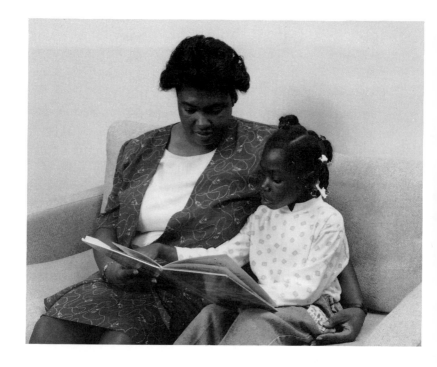

Worksheet for Figuring Your Indexed Earnings

A	B	C		D	E	F
Calendar Year	Maximum Taxable Amount	Enter Your Taxable Earnings	×	Index Factor	= Indexed Earnings	High Years
1951	$ 3,600			8.48595		
1952	3,600			7.98889		
1953	3,600			7.56617		
1954	3,600			7.52733		
1955	4,200			7.19490		
1956	4,200			6.72455		
1957	4,200			6.52261		
1958	4,200			6.46566		
1959	4,800			6.16047		
1960	4,800			5.92783		
1961	4,800			5.81231		
1962	4,800			5.53515		
1963	4,800			5.40266		
1964	4,800			5.19053		
1965	4,800			5.09872		
1966	6,600			4.81000		
1967	6,600			4.55621		
1968	7,800			4.26320		
1969	7,800			4.03028		
1970	7,800			3.83974		
1971	7,800			3.65603		
1972	9,000			3.32972		
1973	10,800			3.13364		
1974	13,200			2.95782		
1975	14,100			2.75214		
1976	15,300			2.57450		
1977	16,500			2.42893		
1978	17,700			2.25023		
1979	22,900			2.06922		
1980	25,900			1.89824		
1981	29,700			1.72463		
1982	32,400			1.63464		
1983	35,700			1.55871		
1984	37,800			1.47217		
1985	39,600			1.41201		
1986	42,000			1.37131		
1987	43,800			1.28910		
1988	45,000			1.22859		
1989	48,000			1.18179		
1990	51,300			1.12962		
1991	53,400			1.08903		
1992	55,500			1.03567		
1993	57,600			1.02684		
1994	60,600			1.00000		
1995	61,200			1.00000		
1996	62,700			1.00000		

Note: Index factors change each year based on U.S. average wage.

Example — Survivor Benefits

In 1996, John dies at age 45, leaving five survivors. Each family member is entitled to a monthly benefit based on John's PIA of $800, as shown below:

Survivor	Qualification for Benefit	Percent of John's PIA	Unadjusted Monthly Benefit Amounts
Mary	Wife, age 45, caring for child under age 16	75	$ 600
Bob	Age 18, in high school	75	600
Suzanne	Age 15	75	600
Bruce	Age 11	75	600
Ruth	John's dependent mother, age 75	82½	660
		Total	$3,060

In the case of John's family, the Maximum Family Benefit is $1,494 (see table on pages 84-85). This means that everyone's benefit must be reduced proportionately so that the total doesn't go over that amount.

Adjusted Monthly Benefit Amounts

Mary	$ 292
Bob	292
Suzanne	292
Bruce	292
Ruth	326
Total	$1,494

Bob Graduates from High School

When Bob graduates from high school at age 18, he is no longer eligible for Social Security benefits. His monthly benefit of $292 stops. However, the rest of the family continues to receive the same total benefit. From the total original entitlement of $3,060, subtract $600 for Bob, leaving $2,460. That's still larger than the Maximum Family Benefit of $1,494. The total stays the same, but each person's check will now be for a different amount.

Readjusted Benefits after Bob Graduates

Mary	$ 364
Suzanne	364
Bruce	364
Ruth	402
Total	$1,494

Bruce Reaches Age 16

Mary's benefit as a mother caring for an eligible child stops when Bruce reaches age 16. (Suzanne is ineligible by then because she is over age 18.) However, Bruce remains entitled to a benefit until he is 18 (or until 19 if he is still in high school). Ruth's benefit also continues. The family's total benefit becomes:

Bruce	$ 600
Ruth	660
Total	$1,260

Bruce Reaches Age 18

When the youngest child reaches age 18 and has completed high school, all the children's benefits will have stopped. Ruth died last year. No further benefits are payable until Mary reaches age 60, unless she becomes disabled and qualifies as a disabled surviving spouse.

Mary at Age 60 in 2011

Mary can claim a surviving spouse's benefit of $572 a month for the rest of her life. That amount is $71\frac{1}{2}\%$ of John's PIA of $800. Or, she can wait until she reaches her Normal Retirement Age of 66 to start receiving her benefit which will then be $800 per month. If she works after her benefits begin, she is subject to the Earnings Limitation (pages 60-64).

Mary at Age 66 in 2017

If Mary waits until she is 66 before receiving benefits, she will receive 100% of John's PIA, or $800 a month. The Earnings Limitation continues to apply until age 70.

8

Medicare

Two Parts of Medicare

The Medicare program has two parts. Part A is Hospital Insurance. Part B is Supplementary Medical Insurance.

Part A of Medicare pays some of the costs of hospitalization, certain related inpatient care, skilled nursing facility care, and home health services. Part B primarily covers doctors' fees, most outpatient hospital services, and certain related services.

Part A is financed primarily by payroll taxes based on covered work, both before and after becoming eligible for benefits. About one-fourth of the cost of Part B is financed by monthly premiums from those who enroll in the program and about three-fourths by the general revenues of the federal government.

Part A benefits are provided automatically on the basis of past work. Part B benefits are available only if you pay the monthly premiums — and about 95% of those eligible do.

When It's Available

Medicare becomes available at the beginning of the month in which you turn 65, whether you are retired or still working. Medicare may also be available if you are disabled, or if you have chronic kidney disease (page 103). Certain of your family members with kidney disease may also qualify.

You automatically apply for Medicare when you apply for Social Security benefits. When you become entitled to Medicare, Social Security will ask you if you wish to enroll in Part B or decline it. If you plan to work past age 65, you should apply for Medicare separately when you turn 65. Your spouse can qualify for Part A of Medicare at age 65 based on **your** work record if you are **eligible** for monthly Social Security benefits, even if you are not yet 65. Almost everyone in the U.S. can enroll in Part B at age 65; they must pay the monthly premium (pages 108-109).

Hospital Insurance (Part A)

Who Can Get Hospital Insurance Benefits

You are eligible for benefits under Part A of Medicare if you are age 65 or over and are eligible for any type of monthly Social Security or Railroad Retirement benefit. Such eligibility can be for benefits as a retired worker, as a spouse of a retired or disabled worker, or as a surviving spouse of a deceased worker. Even if you are not eligible in one of the ways described, you can be eligible on the basis of government employment on which you or your spouse paid the Medicare payroll tax. There is no eligibility for people who receive monthly benefits solely on the basis of one of the international agreements on Social Security that the U.S. has with several countries (see page 158).

You can qualify even if you do not receive monthly Social Security benefits because you or your spouse continues to work.

You should contact the Social Security Administration to apply for your Medicare card about three months before you become 65. This is not necessary if you are already receiving monthly benefits. Even if you don't claim retirement benefits, you should apply for Part A. However, if you don't and are hospitalized, you can still receive benefits retroactively for up to six months when you apply.

If you are disabled, you may be eligible for Medicare Part A before age 65. You must have been entitled to disability benefits from Social Security for at least two years as a worker, surviving spouse, or adult child of a retired disabled or deceased worker. You don't have to apply for a Medicare card in this event; enrollment in such cases is automatic. Family members of disabled workers are not eligible for Medicare benefits before age 65 unless they have been entitled to monthly benefits because of their own disability for at least two years.

Special provisions for Part A coverage apply to people with chronic kidney disease who require dialysis or a transplant. In such cases, you are eligible for Part A at any age if you are an insured worker or the spouse or dependent child of an insured worker (including survivors of a deceased insured worker). You must apply for this Part A coverage.

What Do You Pay for Hospital Insurance

Some of the payroll taxes that employees and employers pay are for Part A of Medicare. Certain government employees who are not under Social Security pay the Medicare tax and receive credits toward Part A benefit coverage. Included are federal employees hired before 1984 and state and local government employees hired after March 1986. The tax is paid on all annual earnings at a tax rate of 1.45%. Self-employed persons pay twice this rate — 2.90%. No taxes or premiums are required for this insurance after you stop working.

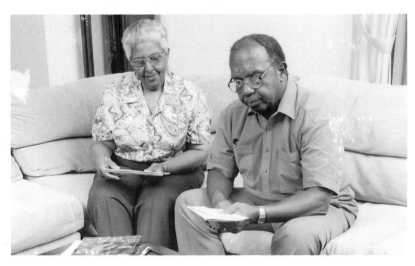

Special rules apply to uninsured people who are at least age 65 but not eligible for Part A under the regular rules. People born before 1903 usually have Part A coverage regardless of their Social Security coverage or eligibility. Other uninsured people can purchase Part A coverage by paying substantial premiums. In 1996, the standard Part A monthly premium for uninsured persons, who are not otherwise eligible for premium-free Part A, is $289. This is reduced to $188 for uninsured persons who have at least 30 credits. They must also enroll in Part B and pay a monthly premium for that coverage (page 109). Disabled people who lose their cash benefits because they returned to work can continue under Medicare for up to 36 months; after that time, they can purchase Medicare in the same way as uninsured people age 65 or over.

What Benefits Does Hospital Insurance Provide
In addition to the basic benefits for inpatient hospital care, Part A provides benefits for skilled nursing facility care, home health services, and hospice care. In most cases, you must pay part of the costs of covered services. Some people carry additional private insurance — Medicare supplement policies (pages 131-141) — to cover some or all of the costs that Medicare doesn't cover. Medicare covers only services that are medically necessary, and it limits the charges to certain allowable amounts.

The amounts that you pay change each year, depending on increases in hospital costs. The following description is based on 1996 amounts, which will increase again next year.

Hospital Benefits. When you are admitted to a hospital, you will have to pay an initial deductible of $736, but no more than the actual charges. For the 61st through the 90th day, you will have to pay $184 per day. After that, you can choose to pay $368 per day for up to 60 "lifetime reserve" days (instead of paying what the hospital charges). Your "benefit period" ends 60 days after discharge from a hospital or skilled nursing facility. If another hospital admission occurs after that, you will have to pay another deductible, as well as the coinsurance (cost-sharing) amounts described above. Appliances such as pacemakers and artificial limbs that are permanently installed while in the hospital are covered without further cost sharing.

Skilled Nursing Facility Benefits. You may qualify for limited benefits at a skilled nursing facility if both the facility and your diagnosis and treatment plan meet Medicare's strict standards. Daily skilled nursing or rehabilitation services must be available to you. Custodial care is not provided. Skilled nursing facility benefits are available to you only following a hospital stay of at least three days and beginning within 30 days of leaving the hospital.

If you qualify, you pay nothing for the first 20 days, except for any charges that Medicare does not allow. For the next 80 days, you pay charges up to $92 per day, and Medicare pays all remaining allowable charges. No benefits are available after 100 days of care in a "benefit period."

Home Health Services Benefits. Home health services, such as part-time or intermittent skilled nursing care, physical therapy, medical social services, medical supplies, and some rehabilitation equipment, may be paid for in full by Medicare when you are confined at home, as long as the services are prescribed by a doctor. You are **not** required to have a hospital stay before home health services are covered. Services must be provided by a home health agency that participates in Medicare.

Hospice Benefits. A hospice is an organization that furnishes a coordinated program of inpatient, outpatient, and home care for terminally ill patients. Emphasis is on counseling, control of symptoms, and pain reduction, but not curative treatment. When you are an inpatient in a facility (not to exceed five consecutive days), in order to provide respite for your usual caretaker, you pay 5% of this cost. Also you pay 5% of the cost for prescription drugs, but not more than $5 for each prescription, for symptom management and pain relief. Hospice benefits are limited to 210 days unless you are recertified as terminally ill. When you choose hospice benefits, all other Medicare benefits stop, except for physician services and treatment of conditions not related to the terminal illness.

Care in Christian Science Sanatoriums. Part A of Medicare can help pay for inpatient hospital and skilled nursing facility services that you receive in a Christian Science sanatorium operated or listed and certified by First Church of Christ Scientist in Boston.

Care in Psychiatric Hospitals. Part A will pay for up to 190 days of inpatient psychiatric care in a lifetime. Restrictions apply to people who are hospitalized for psychiatric care when they are first covered by Medicare.

Care in Non-Participating Hospitals. A few qualified hospitals do not participate in the Medicare program. Medicare will pay part or, in some cases, all of your expenses in a non-participating hospital if you have an emergency, and it is the closest hospital.

Blood Deductible. Part A will pay for inpatient blood transfusions, except for the first three pints per year. You cannot be charged for the first three pints of blood that you replace, or if the blood is part of the deductible under Part B.

Diagnosis Related Groups

To avoid excessive hospital stays, Medicare pays fixed amounts to hospitals for inpatient care, according to diagnosis. But your doctor still decides when you are ready to go home.

Supplementary Medical Insurance (Part B)
Who Can Get Supplementary Medical Insurance Benefits

When you enroll in Part A of Medicare, you also automatically enroll in Part B, unless you tell the Social Security Administration that you don't want it. This procedure applies to people age 65 or older, long-term disabled beneficiaries, and people with chronic kidney disease. Even if you are not eligible for premium-free Part A (see pages 102-104), you can almost always enroll in Part B at age 65. A general enrollment period (January through March each year) is available for persons who did not elect Part B when first eligible.

What Do You Pay for Supplementary Medical Insurance

If you enroll in Part B at the earliest opportunity, you pay premiums of $42.50 per month during 1996. These premiums, which pay only about one-fourth of the cost of Part B, are ordinarily deducted from your Social Security benefits, if you get them. Otherwise, you will be billed by the government quarterly in advance. The monthly premiums are adjusted every January.

If you enroll late, or if you drop out and enroll again, you may have to pay higher premiums. You will pay 10% more for each full 12 months that you were eligible but did not participate. You don't include in such 12-month periods any months when you weren't enrolled in Part B while an active employee, or spouse of an active employee, covered by an employer-sponsored group insurance plan (page 117). Coverage under Part B can begin immediately when your group coverage as an active employee or spouse of an active employee ends. You get a special seven-month enrollment period beginning with the month when coverage ends, or when your active-employee status ends.

What Benefits Does Supplementary Medical Insurance Provide

You pay the first $100 of charges **allowable** by Medicare for covered medical services provided to you in a calendar year. This is the annual deductible. After that, you will pay 20% of covered expenses (which may not exceed the charges allowed by Medicare) plus any additional amount that the physician is **allowed** to charge (see pages 115-116). The Medicare program covers only services that are medically necessary.

The annual deductible of $100 and the 20% patient coinsurance charge do not apply to certain payments (page 111).

Covered items are:

- physician services, regardless of where provided, and supplies furnished as part of such services;
- physical therapy, speech pathology, and occupational therapy by physicians or institutional providers, including comprehensive outpatient rehabilitation facilities;
- services of independent physical therapists and occupational therapists, but with limits (page 112);
- non-routine vision services by qualified optometrists if they would be covered when performed by a physician;
- diagnostic x-ray, laboratory, and other tests;
- x-ray, radium, and radioactive-isotope therapy (including technician services);
- periodic mammography screening;
- flu shots and pneumococcal vaccine;
- blood for transfusions, after the first three pints per year (including any considered under Part A);
- drugs that cannot be self-administered, blood-clotting factors for hemophilia, certain oral anti-cancer drugs, injectable osteoporosis drugs, and immunosuppressive drugs used during the first year after an organ transplant;
- surgical dressings, splints, casts, and similar medical supplies ordered by a doctor;
- necessary ambulance services;
- rental of durable medical equipment used in the home, including oxygen tanks, hospital beds, and wheelchairs (under some circumstances, purchase of such equipment);
- home health services (the same as provided by Part A) for persons who are enrolled in Part B only;

- artificial replacements for parts of the body (covered by Part A under some circumstances);
- colostomy bags and supplies; and
- braces for limbs, back, or neck.

Here are some special provisions:

Services Covered with No Cost-Sharing. You do not have to pay the $100 deductible or the 20% coinsurance for:

- pneumococcal vaccine and flu shots and the charge for giving them;
- outpatient clinical diagnostic laboratory tests performed by physicians (who **must** take assignment for such tests), by independent laboratories that are Medicare-certified, by certified hospitals (except in Maryland, where 20% coinsurance is applicable), and by rural health clinics;
- home health services.

Part B helps to pay for only one type of treatment by licensed and Medicare-certified **chiropractors:** manual manipulation of the spine to correct a subluxation (vertebrae out of place) that can be demonstrated by x-ray. Medicare does not pay for the x-ray or for any other diagnostic or therapeutic services furnished by chiropractors.

Outpatient treatment of **mental illness** is covered under special payment rules. You will ordinarily pay 50% of allowable charges. However, you will pay only 20% of allowable outpatient hospital charges if you would have required admission to the hospital without the treatment. Also, you will pay any additional amount that the physician is **allowed** to charge (see pages 115-116).

Part B does not ordinarily pay for routine foot care, such as hygienic care, treatment for flat feet or other structural misalignment, or removal of calluses, corns, and most warts. It will help to pay for other services of a podiatrist, including routine care if the patient has a condition affecting the lower limbs such as severe diabetes.

Services of independent **physical therapists** and **occupational therapists** are covered. Medicare pays up to a maximum of $720 per year (80% × $900) for each type.

Special reimbursement provisions apply to services rendered by **Health Maintenance Organizations (HMOs)** and similar forms of prepaid medical care that provide a broader scope of benefits than does Medicare. If the HMO's financial experience is favorable, one or more of the following benefits will be provided to Medicare participants: elimination or reduction of the Medicare coinsurance provisions; additional benefits (such as physical exams and eye care); or lower dues to the organization.

People who elect **hospice** benefits have certain restrictions — and also extra benefits (page 107).

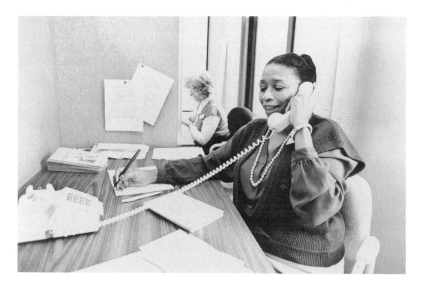

What Medicare Does Not Cover

Medicare does not cover all healthcare expenses. A telephone call to the carrier that handles your Medicare claim is the best way to get answers to your questions about specific cases. Some of the items not covered are:

- services not reasonable or medically necessary;
- items or services for which you are not legally obligated to pay;
- services paid for by the government or workers' compensation;
- services performed by a relative or household member;
- services outside the U.S. (exceptions are Canadian and Mexican facilities if they are nearest to your home or while you are traveling to or from Alaska through Canada);
- routine physical exams;
- routine eye exams and glasses;
- hearing aids;

- dental services (except surgery on, or reduction of, any fracture of the jaw or facial bones);
- routine foot care and orthopedic shoes except for diabetics (page 112);
- custodial care;
- cosmetic surgery (except after an accident);
- most prescription drugs and medicines taken at home;
- acupuncture;
- most immunizations;
- first three pints of blood for transfusions (each year);
- meals delivered to your home;
- private nurses;
- extra charges for a private room (unless medically necessary), telephone, television, and other personal comfort items;
- homemaker services (except under hospice respite provisions);
- certain services for employees and their family members who have primary coverage under employer-provided healthcare plans (pages 116-123);
- certain services in the first 18 months of treatment for chronic kidney disease when covered by an employer-provided healthcare plan; and
- certain services covered by liability or automobile insurance.

Claim Number

When you become eligible for Medicare benefits, you will receive a Medicare card containing your claim number. This number is very important to keep because no claim will be paid without it. The card is the only evidence that you are covered by Medicare.

How Claims Are Paid

Claims are processed by an "intermediary" (Part A) or a "carrier" (Part B). These are insurance companies or other organizations, such as Blue Cross/Blue Shield, under contract to the government. Check your last claim form for the name and address of the carrier. (See pages 142-147 for the names and telephone numbers of Medicare carriers.)

Hospital charges to be paid by Medicare are billed by the hospital to the intermediary that pays them.

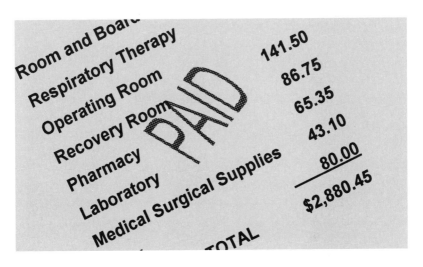

Room and Board	141.50
Respiratory Therapy	86.75
Operating Room	65.35
Recovery Room	43.10
Pharmacy	
Laboratory	
Medical Surgical Supplies	80.00
TOTAL	$2,880.45

Doctors and other suppliers of covered medical services may submit charges directly to the Medicare carrier by "taking an assignment." Your doctor will receive the portion of the bill paid by Medicare and will bill you only for your $100 deductible, if any, and 20% coinsurance payment. Doctors and suppliers who take assignments may not charge more than the amount allowable by Medicare.

Even if the doctor does not take assignment, he or she must send the claim to the Medicare carrier for you. Medicare will pay you on the portion of the bill that is allowable, and you will have to pay the doctor directly. Some charges may be higher than those allowable by Medicare, but the doctor cannot charge more than 15% above the allowable charge. Because your benefit payment will be based on the allowable charge, you will have to pay the excess over the allowable charge, the $100 deductible if not already paid, and the 20% coinsurance.

Coordination with Other Plans

If you are eligible for Medicare benefits and are neither working with employer-sponsored healthcare coverage of an employer with 20 or more employees, nor married to a working person with such coverage, then Medicare is your "primary payer." In that case, Medicare ordinarily pays your medical bills before any other insurance coverage. The other insurance plan, if any, is your "secondary payer," paying whatever benefits are required by it after Medicare pays.

Medicare As Secondary Payer Under Part A

If you are eligible for Medicare benefits at age 65 or older and are working for an employer with 20 or more employees, then you are entitled to the same employer-sponsored healthcare coverage offered to younger employees. If you have such coverage and are working, then Medicare is the secondary payer, paying only with respect to charges not covered by your employer-provided plan. These same rules apply to your spouse at age 65 or older with respect to coverage under your plan, if you are working for such an employer, regardless of your age. These rules also apply to any disabled Medicare enrollee who is also covered by an employer-provided healthcare plan as a currently working employee or as a family member of an employee. However, this applies only if the plan covers employees of at least one employer with 100 or more employees. In those cases where the "size of firm" condition is not met, Medicare is the primary payer, and the plan is secondary.

Under any of these circumstances, you may choose not to participate in Part B of Medicare and thus not pay the monthly premiums. Or else you may choose not to participate in the employer-provided plan, in which case you will have Medicare coverage only.

Medicare is also the secondary payer when medical care can be paid for under any liability policy, such as automobile insurance.

The rules for paying claims when Medicare is secondary are complex, but they follow the general practice in private health insurance plans when the primary/secondary situation exists.

For hospital bills under Part A, Medicare pays the **smaller** of (1) what would have been paid if Medicare were primary, or (2) the Medicare-allowable charge, minus what the other plan actually pays. Consider a patient who has not previously met the Part A deductible and is hospitalized in 1996, with billed charges of $2,000 and a Medicare-allowable charge of $1,600. The other plan, which has a $100 deductible and 20% coinsurance, pays $1,520 (80% of: $2,000 minus $100). If Medicare were primary, it would pay the hospital $864 ($1,600, minus the $736 deductible). Thus, the second alternative, which is smaller, is the amount paid to the hospital: $80 ($1,600, minus the $1,520 benefit under the plan).

If the other plan provided a benefit of $1,600 or more, then Medicare would pay nothing. But if it paid less than $736, then Medicare would pay $864 to the hospital (the allowable charge, minus the deductible), and the patient would pay the difference between the $736 deductible and the other plan's benefit.

In summary, the hospital always receives (from the plan, Medicare, and/or the patient) at least as much as the Medicare-allowable charge. The hospital receives more **only** when the other plan's benefit **alone** is more. The patient will usually pay nothing or, at most, only part of the Part A deductible. Even when the individual has no liability, the deductible is met for any subsequent hospitalization in that "benefit period."

Medicare As Secondary Payer Under Part B
For doctors' bills under Part B, Medicare's payment as the secondary payer depends on whether the doctor takes assignment. In the absence of assignment, when Medicare is the secondary payer, its payment for physician services is the **smaller** of (1) what Medicare would pay if it were primary, (2) the actual charge, minus what the other plan pays, or (3) the higher of the Medicare-allowable charge or the other plan's allowable charge, minus what the plan pays (both charges are without regard to any coinsurance payments).

Continuing with the non-assignment situation, consider a private plan that requires a 20% coinsurance payment and assume that both the $100 Part B deductible and any deductible under the private plan have been met. Assume that the plan's allowable charge is $180, and Medicare's allowable charge is $160, and the physician's bill is the maximum that Medicare will permit, $184 (i.e., 115% of $160). Calculations must be made using the three methods:

(1) In the absence of the other plan, Medicare would pay $128 (80% of $160).

(2) The actual charge of $184, minus the $144 (80% of $180), that the plan would pay in the absence of Medicare, equals $40.

(3) The plan's allowable charge of $180 (which is **higher** than Medicare's allowable charge of $160), minus the $144 that the plan pays, equals $36.

The Medicare payment is $36, the smallest of the three amounts calculated. The second method is rarely used — only when the actual charge is less than the plan's allowable charge.

If the physician takes assignment, then Medicare pays the **smaller** of (1) what it would pay if it were primary, or (2) the Medicare-allowable charge, minus what the other plan pays. Calculations must be made using the two methods:

(1) In the absence of the other plan, Medicare pays $128 (80% of $160).

(2) The Medicare-allowable charge ($160), minus the payment of the plan (80% of $180, or $144), equals $16.

The Medicare payment is $16, the smaller of the two amounts. Method 2 is generally used — except when the Medicare deductible of $100 had not been met, or when the benefit under the other plan is very small. The underlying principle is that Medicare will not pay an amount that would result in the total of all benefits paid exceeding the Medicare allowable charge.

As another example of an assigned physician claim, suppose that this is the first expense of the year. If the Medicare-allowable charge is $160, and the plan's benefit is $60, then Method 1 gives $48 (80% of: $160 minus $100), and Method 2 gives $100 ($160 minus $60). The Medicare benefit is $48, the smaller amount. The Part B deductible is satisfied for the remainder of the year.

Medicare Primary/Secondary Rules as Related To Employer-Provided Health Benefits[1]

(For employees of firms with 20 or more employees)

Category of Individual	Individual	Non-employed Spouse 65 or Over[2]	Spouse Under 65	Disabled Child[3]
I. Employee age 65 or over	Medicare is secondary[4]	Medicare is secondary[4,5]	No Medicare[7,9]	Medicare is secondary[4,5,9]
II. Employee age 62-64	No Medicare[6]	Medicare is secondary[4,5]	No Medicare[7,9]	Medicare is secondary[4,5,9]
III. Employee under age 62	No Medicare[6]	No Part A Medicare unless on own work record or voluntarily purchased, and Part B only if purchased; Medicare coverage when having Part A on own work record, whether or not having Part B, is secondary[4,10]	No Medicare[7,9]	No Medicare[7,9]
IV. Retiree age 65 or over	Medicare is primary	Medicare is primary	No Medicare[7]	Medicare is primary
V. Retiree age 62-64	No Medicare[7,8]	Medicare is primary	No Medicare[7]	Medicare is primary
VI. Retiree under age 62	No Medicare[7,8]	No Part A Medicare unless (a) based on own work record, (b) voluntarily purchased, or (c) the retired spouse receives Social Security disability benefits; Part B only if purchased; Medicare is primary	No Medicare[7]	No Part A Medicare unless the retired parent receives Social Security disability benefits; Part B only if purchased; Medicare is primary[8]

1. Assumes that individuals always file for Part A (Hospital Insurance), if eligible. For both employees and spouses, if Medicare Part B (Supplementary Medical Insurance) is waived because of good coverage of employer plan and to avoid paying the premiums ($42.50 per month in 1996), then such plan is primary. When employment ends (or, if earlier, when coverage under employer plan is ended or, for the disabled, when such plan is no longer primary to Medicare), the individual is eligible for a special enrollment period, and the Medicare Part B premium surcharge for delayed enrollment is waived even though the employer has fewer than 20 employees, in which case Medicare is always primary.) (Such surcharge waiver applies even though the employer has fewer than 20 employees, in which case Medicare is always primary.)

2. If spouse is aged 65 or over and is employed and covered under own employer's plan (with 20 or more employees), Medicare is secondary in any event (subject to footnote 4).

3. Receiving disabled-child benefits (based on becoming disabled before age 22) for at least 24 months after attainment of age 18, and not employed (if employed, and covered under own employer's plan subject to footnote 8; Medicare is secondary in any event — subject to footnote 4). The attendance of the disabled child at high school at age 18 (and before age 19) does not affect the running of such 24-month period.

4. Unless employer plan is waived.

5. Assumes that worker is eligible for retirement benefits (even though not receiving them because of earned income level).

6. Unless disabled and in a rehabilitation trial work period (and also in the following three months and in a further 36 months if engaging in substantial gainful employment even though not medically recovered) and meets (or had met) conditions of footnotes 7 and 8.

7. Unless, on basis of own work record, Social Security disability benefits are being received and have been received for 24 months or more.

8. For plans covering employees of at least one employer with 100 or more employees, Medicare is secondary for a disabled employee who qualifies for Social Security disability benefits and has received such payments for 24 months, but only if the disabled employee is considered to be a currently working employee; otherwise for such disabled former employees, Medicare is primary.

9. For plans covering employees of at least one employer with 100 or more employees, Medicare is secondary for the disabled spouse or child of an employee if such person, on the basis of his or her own work record, qualifies for Social Security disability benefits and has received such payments for 24 months, providing that the spouse or child is covered under the employer plan as a dependent of the employee.

10. If has only Part B, or if has Part A voluntarily purchased (and, therefore, must have Part B), then Medicare is primary.

123

Examples — Part B Monthly Premiums

Mr. Allen took early-retirement cash benefits under Social Security when he reached age 63 in May 1994. On May 1, 1996, the beginning of the month he turns 65, he is automatically covered by Medicare Part A and Part B. Part A coverage was earned while Mr. Allen was working; no monthly premiums are required. Monthly premiums are required for Part B coverage, but he can refuse it if he does not want to pay the premiums. If he takes no action, the monthly premiums for Part B will be automatically deducted from his Social Security benefits, beginning with the benefit payable on May 3, which deduction is the premium for that month. The standard Part B monthly premium in 1996 is $42.50.

Ms. Evans was working and had substantial wages when she turned 65 in 1996. She informed the Social Security Administration that she wanted to enroll in Medicare Part B. Enrollment in Part B results in automatic coverage under Part A. She could have applied for only Part A if she did not want to pay the Part B premiums. The government bills her for her Part B coverage. When she retires and begins to receive monthly Social Security benefits, the monthly premiums will be automatically deducted from her benefits.

Mr. Garcia retired at age 65 in March 1993 and began receiving Social Security benefits. He decided not to enroll in Part B then because he believed that he was in excellent health and saw no reason to pay the premiums. Later, he decides that coverage would be desirable — especially because he would be paying far less than the value of the Part B protection (page 109). He can enroll during the first three months of 1996, with coverage beginning July 1. At that time, he will have been eligible for, but not participating in, Part B for more than three years but less than four years. Therefore, his monthly premiums will be 30% higher than the standard rate for the rest of his life, or $55.20 per month in 1996.

Example — Medicare Benefits for Physician Visits

Mr. Allen, age 72, has acute arthritis and visits his physician, Dr. Williams, every two months for continued observation of his condition and for review of the effect of the drugs that he is taking. Dr. Williams is a "participating physician" (one who always takes assignment) and sends the bills to the Medicare carrier that handles Part B claims. Dr. Williams usually charges $47 for office visits, plus varying amounts for tests made by an outside laboratory. Medicare allows only $40 for the office visits, and so Dr. Williams can charge Mr. Allen only this amount. Medicare pays the entire allowed amount of the laboratory-test bills. This amount is not necessarily what the laboratory would charge a non-Medicare patient, but rather is a rate set by Medicare.

Mr. Allen pays Dr. Williams $80 for the first two visits in 1996. The Medicare carrier allows all of this amount and applies it to Mr. Allen's annual deductible of $100. After Dr. Williams submits a $40 bill for Mr. Allen's third visit in the year, the Medicare carrier sends Mr. Allen a statement showing that the total allowable charges for the year are $120, so that the $100 deductible is met. The carrier also sends Dr. Williams a check for $16, which is 80% of $20 ($120 minus $100). Mr. Allen is responsible for paying Dr. Williams the remainder of the allowable charges of $120 directly. For subsequent visits, Medicare pays a benefit of $32 (80% of $40) to Dr. Williams, and Mr. Allen must pay him the remaining $8.

The laboratory bills Medicare directly, and Mr. Allen receives only a notice of the payments made for the services rendered.

If Dr. Williams **did not** always accept assignment as a participating physician, the situation would be quite different. For non-participating physicians, Medicare's allowable charges are 5% lower than in participating-physician cases. Thus, under these circumstances, the allowable charge for each visit would be $38 (95% of $40). Dr. Williams cannot bill Mr. Allen for more than $43.70 (115% of $38), even though his usual charge is $47. He would, as required by law, send the bills to the Medicare carrier and would bill Mr. Allen what Medicare will allow — $43.70 for each visit. After the first three visits in 1996, Medicare would tell Mr. Allen that the deductible was met, because the total allowable charges then amounted to $114, and would send him a check for $11.20 (80% of: $114 minus the $100 deductible). For each subsequent visit, Medicare would pay Mr. Allen $30.40 (80% of $38). At the same time, Mr. Allen would pay Dr. Williams $43.70 for each visit.

If Dr. Williams made the laboratory tests himself, instead of sending them to an independent laboratory, the reimbursement procedure would depend on whether he takes assignments for such tests, regardless of whether he takes assignments for other services. If he takes assignments for the tests, he would submit the bill to the Medicare carrier and receive the full allowable charge from Medicare, in accordance with a Medicare schedule, and not his usual charge. Mr. Allen would pay nothing. However, if Dr. Williams did not take assignments for such tests, Medicare would not pay anything.

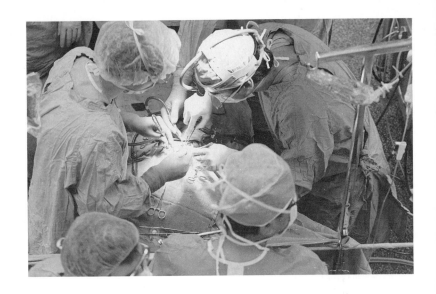

Example — Medicare Benefits for Hospitalization

Mrs. Brown, age 67, broke her hip in February 1996 and was taken to the hospital. The surgeon had to install a prosthetic hip joint. For the patient's own convenience, a private nurse was hired to stay with her at the hospital on the first day after the surgery. She moved from this hospital after seven days to a skilled nursing home for four days, where she received therapy. After returning home, she still needed a physical therapist and a nurse for some treatments, as well as a wheelchair and hospital bed.

Mrs. Brown had previously paid the $100 Part B deductible for earlier expenses. Medicare paid $4,659. She (or her other insurance) had to pay the remaining $1,841.

Because the charges for the doctors and for certain other services were higher than the allowable charges for the same services in her area, only the lower charges were allowed for Medicare reimbursement.

Her charges are itemized below, along with the amounts paid by various parties:

Expenses	Charges	Medicare Allowed	Medicare Paid	Balance Due
Ambulance to hospital	$ 75	$ 70[a]	$ 56[b]	$ 19
Hospital	3,660[c]	3,445	2,709[d]	951
Anesthesiologist	345	300[a]	240[b]	105
Surgeon	1,265	1,100[a]	880[b]	385
Private nurse	120	0[e]	0[e]	120
Ambulance to nursing home	75	70[a]	56[b]	19
Skilled nursing home	400[f]	360	360	40
Ambulance to residence	75	70[a]	56[b]	19
Rental, wheelchair	50	40[a]	32[b]	18
Rental, hospital bed	125	100[a]	80[b]	45
Home visits, therapist	95[g]	95	95	0
Home visits, nurse	95[g]	95	95	0
Medicines taken at home	120	0	0	120
Total	$6,500	$5,745	$4,659	$1,841

[a] Actual charge was higher than the customary charge. Doctors and other providers of services did not accept assignments (the allowed charges are 95% of Medicare's standard allowance for doctors who always accept assignment).

[b] Covered by Part B — 80% paid.

[c] This amount is not technically a "charge." It is Medicare's allowance for Mrs. Brown's diagnosis (which is lower than the usual charges for a non-Medicare, individually-paying patient), plus the costs for luxury items that Medicare does not cover (in this case, $215 for a private room and TV rental).

[d] Exclusive of $736 deductible.

[e] Charges for private nurse are not covered by Medicare.

[f] Includes $40 for TV rental.

[g] Home health agencies must take assignment.

This example shows how helpful Medicare is when you are faced with major expenses. It also shows that you or your other insurance will have to pay some of the expenses.

Fee-For-Service or Managed Care?

Medicare has traditionally operated through the familiar fee-for-service healthcare delivery system described in the preceding pages. Under fee-for-service, the patient chooses the doctor, hospital or other provider of health care. A fee is usually paid each time that a service is received. Medicare determines what it pays, and the patient and/or other insurance are liable for the appropriate charges not paid by Medicare. At present, nearly 90% of persons enrolled in Medicare are under fee-for-service.

Under managed care, services must be obtained only from those doctors, hospitals and other providers who are part of the managed care plan. Managed care plans can take several forms. A Health Maintenance Organization (HMO) is one common type.

Managed care plans combine features of both an insurance company and a healthcare provider. They are similar to an insurance company in that healthcare costs are covered in exchange for payment of a monthly premium. Like other healthcare providers, they perform medical services.

Eligibility to enroll in a managed care plan is available to most Medicare beneficiaries, as long as they are enrolled in Medicare Part B and live within the geographical area that the plan serves.

Although there are restrictions in the choice of doctors and hospitals under managed care plans, there are also a number of advantages, for example:

- lower and more predictable costs for the patient;

- additional services not provided by traditional Medicare, such as physical exams, prescription drugs, dental care, and hearing aids;

- no need for Medigap insurance.

Note, however, even though there is no need for Medigap insurance while you are enrolled in a managed care plan, if you leave it and return to the traditional fee-for-service system, you may be unable to enroll in the Medigap plan of your choice at affordable rates.

Presently only about 10% of persons enrolled in Medicare are in HMOs, but this proportion is likely to increase. First, increasing numbers of persons are joining HMOs during their working careers, and will be accustomed to them when they become eligible for Medicare. Second, HMOs are becoming more available throughout the country. Finally, lawmakers are looking to managed care as an important way to help control escalating costs in the financially troubled Medicare program. Thus, legislation may be enacted that will enable managed care plans to offer additional features, such as increased portability for persons who do not live in the same location throughout the year. Also, the reimbursement procedures used by Medicare to pay providers may eventually make the traditional fee-for-service delivery system less attractive for doctors, hospitals, and other providers and thus become less available for Medicare beneficiaries.

To find out more about managed care plans available in your area call your state insurance counseling office or the Medicare hotline at 1-800-638-6833.

Medicare Supplemental Insurance

Medicare does not pay all of a person's medical expenses. There are deductibles, coinsurance amounts, nonallowable charges, and noncovered services. Most people need additional health insurance to fill the gaps in Medicare.

Many retired persons and their spouses have adequate protection provided by their former employers. Many others purchase Medicare supplement insurance ("Medigap") policies. In the past, when there were many different policies available in the marketplace, knowing which one was best for you was very difficult to determine.

Congress recognized this problem and in 1990 enacted legislation to simplify comparison shopping for Medicare supplement insurance. Since 1992, Medicare supplements have been limited to ten standard plans. One basic plan must be offered in all Medicare supplements. The other nine standard plans offer various features in addition to the basic plan. Not every insurer will offer all ten plans, and all ten plans may not be available in all states.

In addition to the ten standard plans, there is an another option called Medicare Select. This is a preferred provider arrangement in which lower premiums may be charged if the participant agrees to use the services of particular healthcare providers. More detailed information is available from the respective state insurance commissioners. Federal legislation was enacted in 1995 to expand the Medicare Select program to all 50 states. For general information or for the telephone number of your state insurance office, you can call the Medicare hotline at 1-800-638-6833.

The purpose of the 1990 legislation is to standardize the coverage provided by Medicare supplement insurance, to simplify the terms, to eliminate misleading and confusing provisions, and to increase the consumer's understanding of and ability to compare them. The premium cost and, of course, service can vary among the various insurers.

This legislation applies to policies held to be, or marketed as, Medicare Supplement policies. It does not apply to employer or labor union policies for employees or members or for former employees or members.

There are several key provisions in Medicare supplement policies.

(1) No policy can contain benefits that duplicate Medicare benefits.

(2) Newly entitled Medicare Part B beneficiaries who are age 65 or older, have a six-month open enrollment period to purchase such a policy.

(3) No policy can exclude or limit benefits for loss incurred more than six months from the effective date of coverage because it involved a pre-existing condition.

(4) Such policies can provide that benefits which are designed to cover deductibles and coinsurance under Medicare will change automatically as they change under Medicare. Premiums, of course, may be adjusted to correspond with such changes.

(5) States must establish very strict guidelines regarding nonrenewability and cancellation of policies. Generally, policies are not to be canceled or nonrenewed other than for non-payment of premium.

(6) Applicants have the right to return a policy within 30 days of its delivery and receive a refund of the premium if not satisfied for any reason.

The basic benefits included in all standard Medicare supplement plans are:

(1) Coverage of Part A Medicare coinsurance for hospitalization from the 61st day through the 90th day in any Medicare benefit period. This cost is $184 per day in 1996 (page 106);

(2) Coverage of Part A Medicare eligible expenses incurred for hospitalization to the extent not covered by Medicare for each Medicare lifetime inpatient reserve day used. This cost is $368 per day in 1996 (page 106);

(3) Upon exhaustion of the Medicare Part A hospital inpatient coverage, including the lifetime reserve days, coverage of the Medicare Part A eligible expenses for hospitalization, subject to a lifetime maximum benefit of an additional 365 days;

(4) Coverage under Medicare Parts A and B for the reasonable cost of the first three pints of blood (or equivalent quantities of packed red blood cells, as defined under federal regulations) unless replaced in accordance with federal regulations (page 107);

(5) Coverage for the coinsurance amount (20%) of Medicare Part B regardless of hospital confinement, subject to the Medicare Part B deductible of $100 (page 109).

The first Medicare supplement plan, which is designated as Plan A, contains only the basic benefits listed previously.

Each of the remaining nine plans, designated as Plans B through J, also contains the basic benefits plus one or more of the following additional benefits:

(1) Medicare Part A Deductible: Coverage for the Medicare Part A inpatient hospital deductible amount per benefit period, which is $736 in 1996 (page 106).

(2) Skilled Nursing Facility Care: Coverage for the actual billed charges up to the coinsurance amount (charges up to $92 per day in 1996) from the 21st day through the 100th day in a Medicare benefit period for post-hospital skilled nursing facility care eligible under Medicare Part A (page 106).

(3) Medicare Part B Deductible: Coverage for the Medicare Part B deductible of $100 per calendar year, regardless of hospital confinement (page 109).

(4) 80% of the Medicare Part B Excess Charges: Coverage for 80% of the difference between the actual charge as billed (not to exceed any charge limitation established by the Medicare program or state law), and the Medicare allowable Part B charge. (For federal law limits on physician charges for Medicare patients, see page 116.)

(5) 100% of the Medicare Part B Excess Charges: Coverage for all of the difference between the actual charge as billed, (not to exceed any charge limitation established by the Medicare program or state law), and the Medicare-approved Part B charge. (For federal law limits on physician charges for Medicare patients, see page 116.)

(6) Basic Outpatient Prescription Drug Benefit: Coverage for 50% of outpatient prescription drug charges, after a $250 calendar year deductible, to a maximum of $1,250 in benefits received by the insured per calendar year, to the extent not covered by Medicare (page 110).

(7) Extended Outpatient Prescription Drug Benefit: Coverage for 50% of outpatient prescription drug charges, after a $250 calendar year deductible to a maximum of $3,000 in benefits received by the insured per calendar year, to the extent not covered by Medicare (page 110).

(8) Medically Necessary Emergency Care in a Foreign Country: Coverage to the extent not covered by Medicare for 80% of the billed charges for Medicare-eligible expenses for medically necessary emergency hospital, physician,and other medical care received in a foreign country,which care would have been covered by Medicare if provided in the United States, and which care began during the first 60 consecutive days of each trip outside the United States, subject to a calendar year deductible of $250 and a lifetime maximum benefit of $50,000. For such purposes, "emergency care" means care needed immediately because of an injury or an illness of sudden and unexpected onset.

(9) Preventive Medical Care Benefit: Coverage for the following preventive health services:

(a) An annual clinical preventive medical history and physical examination that may include tests and services described in the next paragraph and patient education to address preventive health care measures.

(b) Any one or a combination of the following preventive screening tests or preventive services, as often as medically appropriate:

    (1) fecal occult blood test and/or digital rectal examination;

    (2) mammogram;

    (3) dipstick urinalysis for hematuria, bacteriuria, and proteinauria;

    (4) pure tone (air only) hearing screening test, administered or ordered by a physician;

    (5) serum cholesterol screening (every 5 years);

    (6) thyroid function test; and

    (7) diabetes screening.

(c) Tetanus and diphtheria booster (every 10 years).

(d) Any other tests or preventive measures determined appropriate by the attending physician.

Reimbursement shall be for the actual charges up to 100% of the Medicare-approved amount for each service, as if Medicare were to cover the service as identified in Current Procedural Terminology codes of the American Medical Association, to a maximum of $120 annually for all of the services described above.

(10) At-Home Recovery Benefit: Coverage for services to provide short term, at-home assistance with activities of daily living for those recovering from an illness, injury or surgery.

(a) For purposes of this benefit, the following definitions apply:

(1) "Activities of daily living" include bathing, dressing, personal hygiene, transferring, eating, ambulating, assistance with drugs that are normally self-administered, and changing bandages or other dressings.

(2) "Care provider" means a duly qualified or licensed home health aide/homemaker, personal care aide, or nurse provided through a licensed home health care agency or referred by licensed referral agency or licensed nurses registry.

(3) "Home" shall mean any place used by the insured as a place of residence, provided that such place would qualify as a residence for home health care services covered by Medicare. A hospital or skilled nursing facility shall not be considered the insured's place of residence.

(4) "At-home recovery visit" means the period of a visit required to provide at home recovery care, without limit on the duration of the visit, except that each consecutive 4 hours in a 24-hour period of services provided by a care provider is counted as one visit.

(b) Coverage Requirements and Limitations:

(1) At-home recovery services provided must be primarily services which assist in activities of daily living.

(2) The insured's attending physician must certify that the specific type and frequency of at-home recovery services are necessary because of a condition for which a home care plan of treatment was approved by Medicare.

(3) Coverage is limited to:

(i) no more than the number and type of at-home recovery visits certified as necessary by the insured's attending physician. The total number of at-home recovery visits shall not exceed the number of Medicare-approved home health care visits under a Medicare-approved home care plan of treatment;

(ii) the actual charges for each visit, up to a maximum reimbursement of $40 per visit;

(iii) $1,600 per calendar year;

(iv) seven visits in any week;

(v) care furnished on a visiting basis in the insured's home;

(vi) services provided by a care provider, as defined;

(vii) at-home recovery visits while the insured is covered under the policy or certificate which are not otherwise excluded; and

(viii) at-home recovery visits received during the period that the insured is receiving Medicare-approved home care services or no more than 8 weeks after the service date of the last Medicare-approved home health care visit.

(c) Coverage is excluded for:

(1) home care visits paid for by Medicare or other government programs; and

(2) care provided by family members, unpaid volunteers, or providers who are not "care providers," as defined.

(11) New or Innovative Benefits: An insurer may, with the prior approval of the state commissioner of insurance, offer policies or certificates with new or innovative benefits in addition to the benefits provided in a policy or certificate that otherwise complies with the applicable standards. Such new or innovative benefits may include benefits that are appropriate to Medicare supplement insurance and are new or innovative, not otherwise available, cost-effective, and offered in a manner which is consistent with the goal of simplification of Medicare supplement policies.

The following chart shows what features are in each of the ten standard plans.

Ten Standard Plans

	A	B	C	D	E	F	G	H	I	J
Basic Benefits	✓	✓	✓	✓	✓	✓	✓	✓	✓	✓
Skilled Nursing Coinsurance			✓	✓	✓	✓	✓	✓	✓	✓
Part A Deductible		✓	✓	✓	✓	✓	✓	✓	✓	✓
Part B Deductible			✓			✓				✓
Part B: Percent of Excess Actual Charge over Allowable Charge						100% ✓	80% ✓		100% ✓	100% ✓
Foreign Travel			✓	✓	✓	✓	✓	✓	✓	✓
At-Home Recovery				✓			✓		✓	✓
Basic Drugs ($1,250 limit)								✓	✓	
Extended Drugs ($3,000 limit)										✓
Preventive Care					✓					✓

Medicare Part B Carriers Telephone Numbers

The toll-free or 800 numbers listed below can be used only in the states where the carriers are located.

ALABAMA

Blue Cross-Blue Shield of Alabama

1-800-292-8855
  205-988-2244

ALASKA

Aetna Life Insurance Company

1-800-452-0125
  503-222-6831
    (customer service site in Oregon)

ARIZONA

Aetna Life Insurance Company

1-800-352-0411
  602-861-1968

ARKANSAS

Arkansas Blue Cross and Blue Shield

1-800-482-5525
  501-378-2320

CALIFORNIA

Counties of: Los Angeles, Orange, San Diego, Ventura, Imperial, San Luis Obispo, and Santa Barbara

Transamerica Occidental Life Insurance Company

1-800-675-2266
  213-748-2311

Rest of State

Blue Shield of California

1-800-952-8627
  916-743-1583

COLORADO

Blue Shield of North Dakota

1-800-247-2267
  701-282-0691

CONNECTICUT

The Travelers Companies

1-800-982-6819
  203-728-6783 (In Hartford)
  203-237-8592 (In the Meriden area)

DELAWARE

Xact Medicare Services

1-800-851-3535

DISTRICT OF COLUMBIA

Xact Medicare Services

1-800-233-1124

FLORIDA

Blue Cross and Blue Shield of Florida, Inc.

1-800-333-7586
904-355-3680

GEORGIA

Aetna Life Insurance Company

1-800-727-0827
912-920-2412

HAWAII

Aetna Life Insurance Company

1-800-272-5242
808-524-1240

IDAHO

CIGNA

1-800-627-2782
208-342-7763

ILLINOIS

Health Care Services Corporation

1-800-642-6930
312-938-8000

INDIANA

AdminaStar Federal

1-800-622-4792
317-842-4151

IOWA

IASD Health Services Corporation

1-800-532-1285
515-245-4785

KANSAS

Counties of: Johnson and Wyandotte

Blue Cross and Blue Shield of Kansas, Inc.

1-800-892-5900
816-561-0900

Rest of State

Blue Cross and Blue Shield of Kansas, Inc.

1-800-432-3531
913-232-3773

KENTUCKY

AdminaStar of Kentucky

1-800-999-7608
502-425-6759

LOUISIANA

Arkansas Blue Cross & Blue Shield, Inc.

1-800-462-9666
504-529-1494
(In New Orleans)
504-927-3490
(In Baton Rouge)

MAINE

C and S Administrative Services

1-800-492-0919
   207-828-4300

MARYLAND

Counties of: Montgomery and Prince Georges

Xact Medicare Services

1-800-233-1124

Rest of State

Trail Blazer Enterprises

1-800-492-4795

MASSACHUSETTS

C and S Administrative Services

1-800-882-1228
   617-741-3300

MICHIGAN

HCSC

1-800-482-4045
   313-225-8200

MINNESOTA

Counties of: Anoka, Dakota, Fillmore, Goodhue, Hennepin, Houston, Olmstead, Ramsey, Wabasha, Washington, and Winona

The Travelers Insurance Company

1-800-352-2762
   612-884-7171

Rest of State

Blue Cross and Blue Shield of Minnesota

1-800-392-0343
   612-456-5070

MISSISSIPPI

The Travelers Insurance Company

1-800-682-5417
   601-956-0372

MISSOURI

Counties of: Andrew, Atchison, Bates, Benton, Buchanan, Caldwell, Carroll, Cass, Clay, Clinton, Daviess, DeKalb, Gentry, Grundy, Harrison, Henry, Holt, Jackson, Johnson, Lafayette, Livingston, Mercer, Nodaway, Pettis, Platte, Ray, St. Clair, Saline, Vernon, and Worth

Blue Cross and Blue Shield of Kansas, Inc.

1-800-892-5900
  816-561-0900

Rest of State

General American Life Insurance Company

1-800-392-3070
  314-843-8880

MONTANA

Blue Cross and Blue Shield of Montana, Inc.

1-800-332-6146
  406-444-8350

NEBRASKA

Blue Cross and Blue Shield of Kansas, Inc.

1-800-633-1113

NEVADA

Aetna Life Insurance Company

1-800-528-0311
  602-861-1968

NEW HAMPSHIRE

C and S Administrative Services

1-800-447-1142
  207-828-4300

NEW JERSEY

Xact Medicare Services

1-800-462-9306

NEW MEXICO

Aetna Life Insurance Company

1-800-423-2925
  505-821-3350
     (In Albuquerque)

NEW YORK

Counties of: Bronx, Columbia, Delaware, Dutchess, Greene, Kings, Nassau, New York, Orange, Putnam, Richmond, Rockland, Suffolk, Sullivan, Ulster, and Westchester

Empire Blue Cross and Blue Shield

1-800-442-8430
  516-244-5100

County of: Queens

Group Health, Inc.

212-721-1770

Rest of State

BC/BS of Western New York

1-800-252-6550

NORTH CAROLINA

Connecticut General Life
Insurance Company

1-800-672-3071
  919-665-0348

NORTH DAKOTA

Blue Shield of North Dakota

1-800-247-2267
  701-277-2363

OHIO

Nationwide Mutual Insurance
Company

1-800-282-0530
  614-249-7157

OKLAHOMA

Aetna Life Insurance Company

1-800-522-9079
  405-848-7711

OREGON

Aetna Life Insurance Company

1-800-452-0125
  503-222-6831

PENNSYLVANIA

Xact Medicare Services

1-800-382-1274

RHODE ISLAND

Blue Cross and Blue Shield of
Rhode Island

1-800-662-5170
  401-861-2273

SOUTH CAROLINA

Palmetto Government Benefits
Administrators

1-800-868-2522
  803-788-3882

SOUTH DAKOTA

Blue Shield of North Dakota

1-800-437-4762

TENNESSEE

CIGNA

1-800-342-8900
  615-244-5650

TEXAS

Blue Cross & Blue Shield of
Texas, Inc.

1-800-442-2620
  214-235-3433

UTAH

Blue Shield of Utah

1-800-426-3477
  801-481-6196

VERMONT

C and S Administrative Services

1-800-447-1142
  207-828-4300

VIRGINIA

Counties of: Arlington and Fairfax; Cities of: Alexandria, Falls Church and Fairfax

Xact Medicare Services

1-800-233-1124

Rest of State

The Travelers Insurance Company

1-800-552-3423
  804-330-4786

WASHINGTON

Aetna Life Insurance Company

1-800-372-6604
  206-621-0359 (In Seattle)

WEST VIRGINIA

Nationwide Mutual Insurance Company

1-800-848-0106
  614-249-7157

WISCONSIN

WPS

1-800-944-0051
  608-221-3330 (In Madison)

WYOMING

Blue Cross and Blue Shield of North Dakota

1-800-442-2371
  307-632-9381

AMERICAN SAMOA

Hawaii Medical Services Association

808-944-2247

GUAM

Aetna Life Insurance Company

808-524-1240

NORTHERN MARIANA ISLANDS

Triple-S, Inc.

808-524-1240

PUERTO RICO/VIRGIN ISLANDS

Triple-S, Inc.

1-800-981-7015
      (In Puerto Rico)
  809-749-4900
      (In Puerto Rico metro area)
1-800-474-7448
      (In U. S. Virgin Islands)
  809-774-7915 (In St. Thomas)
  809-773-9548 (In St. Croix)

9

Medicaid

Medicaid is a joint federal and state medical assistance program for persons and families with low incomes and resources. Medicaid was created in 1965 — the same year that Medicare was created. Although the words Medicare and Medicaid sound similar and are often confused with each other, they identify separate programs.

Medicare (pages 101-128) is a federal health insurance program for persons age 65 and over, persons who have been entitled to Social Security disability insurance benefits for at least 24 months, and most persons with kidney failure. Eligibility is closely related to eligibility for Social Security benefits rather than demonstrated financial need.

Medicaid is a means-tested medical assistance program for the poor. It is jointly funded by the federal and state governments. The states administer their own Medicaid programs under federal guidelines. Each state sets its own eligibility requirements, scope of covered medical services, and rates of payments.

Persons eligible for Medicaid include recipients of Aid to Families with Dependent Children (AFDC), most persons receiving Supplemental Security Income (SSI) (pages 172-174), and many nursing home patients after they have exhausted their own funds.

The majority of persons on Medicaid are children and nonelderly adults. The majority of Medicaid expenditures, however, are for the elderly, with most such money paying for nursing home care.

Strict federal guidelines have been enacted in recent years, which are intended to greatly restrict the ability of nursing home patients to transfer their assets to other family members and still qualify for Medicaid. To determine the specific eligibility requirements that exist in your state, contact your state or county Medical Assistance office.

Proposals aimed at curtailing the growth in Medicaid expenditures have recently received much attention in Congress as lawmakers look for ways to balance the federal budget. Those proposals receiving the most attention have called for the federal government to make block grants to the states. This would result in an easing of federal mandates. Proponents argue that this would give the states more discretion to try innovative cost-cutting measures. Critics argue that access to quality care for the poor would be jeopardized. At the time of publication, major legislation in this area has yet to be enacted.

10

Miscellaneous

Social Security Rules

Retirement

(1) Credits needed: Forty credits are required for persons born after 1928. For persons born before 1929, count the number of years **after** 1950 **through** the year you become 61. That's how many **credits** you need to be fully insured and qualified for benefits.

(2) Number of years of earnings needed: Subtract five from the number of credits you need to be fully insured. That's how many years of earnings you must use to figure your Average Indexed Monthly Earnings (AIME).

Disability

(3) Credits needed: Count the number of years **after** you became 21 **through** the year before disability occurs (or **through** the year you become age 61, if earlier). That's how many **credits** you need to be fully insured. To qualify for disability benefits, you must also meet another requirement — 20 credits during the 40 calendar quarters ending with the calendar quarter in which you become disabled. If you do not meet this requirement, then:

(a) If you become disabled at ages 24-31, you need one credit for each two calendar quarters after the time you reached 21 and before the time you become disabled, but not less than 6 credits.

(b) If you become disabled before age 24, you need 6 credits in the 12-quarter period ending with the quarter you become disabled.

(4) Number of years of earnings needed: Subtract a specified number of drop-out years from the number of credits you need to be fully insured for disability on the basis described in the first sentence of item 3. The number of drop-out years is: 0 if you are under age 27 when disabled; 1 for ages 27-31; 2 for ages 32-36; 3 for ages 37-41; 4 for ages 42-46; and 5 for ages 47 or older. The remainder is the number of years of earnings you must use to figure your AIME. The result cannot be less than 2. However, persons disabled before age 37 may have additional child-care drop-out years (page 78).

Death

(5) Credits needed: Count the number of years **after** you became 21 (do not count any year before 1951) **through** the year before death occurs (or **through** the year you become age 61, if earlier). The result cannot be less than 6. That's how many credits you need to be fully insured so that your dependents are qualified for all survivor benefits.

(6) Number of years of earnings needed: Subtract five from the number of credits you need to be fully insured for survivor benefits. The result cannot be less than 2. That's how many years of earnings you must use to figure your AIME.

Primary Insurance Amount (PIA) formula

(7) For persons attaining age 62 in one of the years shown below (or becoming disabled or dying in that year, before age 62), the PIA formula applied to the AIME is:

	PIA Benefit Formula		
Age 62 in	90% of	32% of	15% of
1996	First $437	Next $2,198	Over $2,635
1995	426	2,141	2,567
1994	422	2,123	2,545
1993	401	2,019	2,420
1992	387	1,946	2,333
1991	370	1,860	2,230
1990	356	1,789	2,145
1989	339	1,705	2,044
1988	319	1,603	1,922

To the resulting monthly benefit figure, apply cost-of-living adjustments (COLAs) for the year of attainment of age 62 **and all subsequent years, as follows:**

Year	COLA	Year	COLA
1988	4.0%	1992	3.0%
1989	4.7	1993	2.6
1990	5.4	1994	2.8
1991	3.7	1995	2.6

Note: These COLAs were effective for December and normally payable beginning in January.

The annual cost-of-living adjustment (COLA) for a particular year is determined by comparing price inflation for the third calendar quarter of that year with the same quarter of the previous year. Used for this purpose is the Consumer Price Index for Urban Wage Earners and Clerical Workers (CPI-W).

Maximum Family Benefit (MFB) formula

(8) For persons attaining age 62 in one of the years shown (or dying before age 62 in such year), the MFB formula applied to the PIA is:

Age 62 in	MFB Benefit Formula			
	150% of	272% of	134% of	175% of
1996	First $559	Next $247	Next $246	Over $1,052
1995	544	241	239	1,024
1994	539	240	237	1,016
1993	513	227	226	966
1992	495	219	217	931
1991	473	209	208	890
1990	455	201	200	856
1989	433	193	190	816
1988	407	181	179	767

For disabled persons, the MFB is the smaller of (a) 150% of PIA, or (b) 85% of the AIME, but not less than the PIA. To the resulting monthly benefit figure, apply the appropriate cost-of-living adjustments for subsequent years.

Reduction factors for early retirement

If a benefit begins before age 65, it is reduced as follows:

Worker at ages 62-64 . . . . $5/9$ of 1% for each month below 65

Spouse at ages 62-64 . . . . $25/36$ of 1% for each month below 65

Surviving spouse at ages 60-64 . . . . . $19/40$ of 1% for each month below 65

Disabled surviving spouse
   at ages 50-59 . . . . $28\frac{1}{2}$%

Note: As the Normal Retirement Age (NRA) rises, the factor for the early retirement benefit at age 62 will gradually decline, starting in 2000, from 80% of the Primary Insurance Amount (PIA) to 70% of the PIA. Similarly, a spouse's early retirement benefit at age 62 will gradually change from 75% to 65% of the amount available at the NRA. Reductions will also be larger for surviving spouses first claiming benefits after age 60.

Benefit Eligibility Status for Remarried Spouses

Many persons reaching retirement age have been married more than once. The chart in this section describes what effect, if any, that remarriage has on eligibility for spouse or survivor benefits.

The chart shows the situation for a woman who was married twice — under all possible conditions as to current age, the age at remarriage, and whether or not the husbands involved are still living. **Although the chart relates to women, it is equally applicable to men;** however, few men receive husband's or widower's benefits because the benefit based on their own earnings record is usually larger.

Some of the annotations are marked not applicable (n/a). This is done when the basic eligibility requirements are not met rather than marital status being the relevant factor. Examples: (1) Wife's benefits are not payable before age 62 and (2) Widow's benefits are not payable if the husband is living.

In the case of a woman who had been married more than twice, the chart can be used, in turn, to determine the eligibility status on the basis of each husband's word record by considering the particular ex-husband as "First Husband" and the last husband (or ex-husband) as "Second Husband." For example, in the case of a woman age 68 who had been married three times, with the second remarriage occurring after age 60, and whose first and third husbands are deceased, she is eligible for widow's benefits on the earnings records of both the first and third husbands — according to the last line of the chart — and to divorced wife's benefits on the earnings record of the second husband (if the marriage lasted at least 10 years) — according to the next-to-last line of the chart. She, of course, receives only the largest of such three benefits.

Benefit Eligibility Status for Remarried Woman
(Non-Disabled and Without Eligible Child)
Under Various Conditions

Current Age of Woman	Age at Remarriage	Status of First Husband	Status of Second Husband	Wife's Benefit on		Widow's Benefit on	
				First Husband	Second Husband	First Husband	Second Husband
60-61	Under 60	*	Alive	n/a	n/a	No	n/a
60-61	Under 60	Alive	Dead	n/a	n/a	n/a	Yes
60-61	Under 60	Dead	Dead	n/a	n/a	Yes	Yes
60-61	60+	Alive	Alive	n/a	n/a	n/a	n/a
60-61	60+	Alive	Dead	n/a	n/a	n/a	Yes
60-61	60+	Dead	Alive	n/a	n/a	Yes	n/a
60-61	60+	Dead	Dead	n/a	n/a	Yes	Yes
62+	Under 60	Alive	Alive	No	Yes	n/a	n/a
62+	Under 60	Alive	Dead	Yes	n/a	n/a	Yes
62+	Under 60	Dead	Alive	n/a	Yes	No	n/a
62+	Under 60	Dead	Dead	n/a	n/a	Yes	Yes
62+	60+	Alive	Alive	No	Yes	n/a	n/a
62+	60+	Alive	Dead	Yes	n/a	n/a	Yes
62+	60+	Dead	Alive	n/a	Yes	Yes	n/a
62+	60+	Dead	Dead	n/a	n/a	Yes	Yes

* Regardless of whether alive or dead

Note: Second marriage assumed to terminate only by death. Second marriage assumed to have lasted at least one year. First marriage assumed to have lasted at least 10 years.

Garnishment

Social Security benefits are protected by law from assignment, levy, or garnishment. The only exceptions are: levies by the IRS for unpaid federal taxes, and garnishment orders issued by courts for the enforcement of legal obligations to provide child support or make alimony payments.

Members of the Armed Forces

Members of the armed forces of the U.S. have been covered by Social Security since 1957. They pay taxes on their cash compensation. Further, they receive additional earnings credits of $100 for each $300 of actual earnings, up to a maximum of $1,200 of additional credit per year. (These additional credits were $300 per quarter in 1957-77.) This reflects the value of the food, housing, and clothing that they receive. These additional credits are not always granted if military service is shorter than 2 years.

From 1940 through 1956, military personnel received free earnings credits of $160 per month for periods of service. These credits are not always granted if a federal pension is payable for the same period of service.

Credits that are based on other than actual pay received do not always appear on the Social Security earnings record, but they are used when a benefit application is made, if the credits result in a larger benefit.

Living Outside the U.S.

If you are a Social Security beneficiary, and you live outside of the U.S. for 30 days or more, you must notify the Social Security Administration. This applies even if you have direct deposit of your benefit to a financial institution in the U.S.

The U.S. consists of the 50 states, District of Columbia, American Samoa, Guam, Northern Mariana Islands, Puerto Rico, and U.S. Virgin Islands.

People can usually continue to receive Social Security benefits while living outside the U.S. More restrictive rules apply to persons living outside the U.S. who are not U.S. citizens and are receiving benefits as a dependent or survivor. Social Security will make a determination in each case.

The annual earnings test is replaced with a foreign work test for beneficiaries who work outside the U.S. If you work outside of the U.S. in employment not subject to U.S. Social Security taxes, then work of more than 45 hours a month will cause your benefit to be withheld. There is no limitation once you reach age 70.

If you are neither a U.S. citizen nor a U.S. resident, then 25.5% of your benefit will usually be withheld for federal income tax. This withholding is sometimes reduced or eliminated according to terms of treaties with other countries.

Many foreign countries tax U.S. Social Security benefits. You should contact the embassy in Washington, D.C. of the country in which you plan to live for more information.

Medicare does not cover health services received outside of the U.S., except in very limited circumstances in Canada, and along the U.S. and Mexican border. If you are outside of the U.S. for a long time, you may not want to enroll in or continue Medicare Part B, because of the monthly premium required. However, if you do not enroll, or if you disenroll, there is a premium surcharge of 10 percent per year of nonenrollment if you reenroll later. In such cases, you could reenroll only during the first three months of the year, and coverage would not be effective until the following July (page 109).

International Social Security Agreements

Legislation in 1977 authorized the President to enter into bilateral totalization agreements with other nations for limited coordination of the Social Security program (but not Medicare) with corresponding programs of the other countries. The earnings records of persons who work in the countries with which agreements have been made will be combined for purposes of determining benefit eligibility. Currently, in such agreements, the combination of earnings records is done only for eligibility purposes. When eligibility is obtained **only** because of such totalization, the benefit amount is computed in a special manner.

Another feature of these agreements is that dual simultaneous coverage (and thus dual payment of payroll taxes) will be eliminated. In other words, a citizen of the United States employed in another country by a U.S. employer (and whose coverage under Social Security thus continues) will not be covered under the social insurance system of a nation with which an agreement had been made (as would otherwise have been the case). The same situation, of course, prevails for foreigners working in the United States for an employer of their own country.

Agreements with the following countries are now in effect: Austria, Belgium, Canada, Finland, France, Germany, Greece, Ireland, Italy, Luxembourg, Netherlands, Norway, Portugal, Spain, Sweden, Switzerland, and the United Kingdom. Agreements with other countries are in various stages of negotiation.

Railroad Retirement System

The Social Security program, as indicated previously, covers virtually all nongovernment employment in the United States except for railroad employees, who are covered by the Railroad Retirement system. This separate system is coordinated closely with Social Security, and its general structure is quite similar, although the retirement benefits are significantly higher, and the retirement conditions are somewhat more liberal.

It may be said that Railroad Retirement is a social insurance program, although it has certain characteristics of a large multi-employer, private pension plan. It is administered by the Railroad Retirement Board, with headquarters in Chicago, in conjunction with certain other benefit programs for railroad employees (namely, unemployment insurance and cash sickness benefits).

In order to receive Railroad Retirement benefits, the worker must have at least 10 years of railroad service. If such is not the case, the railroad wages are transferred to Social Security and are counted towards benefits in the usual manner. Railroad Retirement benefits consist of two parts — (1) what is essentially a Social Security benefit and (2) an amount proportionately related to the length of service and the average earnings in the highest 60 months of service.

The conditions for receipt of Railroad Retirement benefits are at least as favorable as under Social Security, and in some instances much more favorable. For example, individuals can retire at age 62 with 30 years of service without the usual reduction for early retirement. Also, disability annuities are available for occupational disability, rather than the strict standards required by Social Security. Further, widowed spouse's benefits are available at age 60, with the reduction for early retirement being only that applicable to retirement at age 62.

Railroad workers and their employers pay exactly the same taxes as do other workers for Social Security and the Hospital Insurance portion of Medicare. They are covered for Medicare just as are all other workers. In addition, in order to finance the more liberal cash benefits, railroad employers pay a tax of 16.1%, and railroad employees pay a tax of 4.9%. The maximum amount on which these taxes are paid is $46,500 in 1996 (which is automatically adjusted each year, in the same manner as is the Social Security maximum taxable amount). Employers also pay a tax of 34 cents per hour that each employee works in January-March 1996 (subject to change each quarter thereafter); this is used to finance supplemental annuities, which amount to $23 to $43 a month.

The Notch

The "Notch" is one of the most misunderstood and controversial Social Security issues in many years. This term refers to a special method of calculating Social Security benefits for people born in 1917-21, the result of legislation enacted in 1977. Nineteen years later, this issue is still in the forefront of public debate on Social Security. These "notch babies" believe that they are receiving less favorable benefit treatment than those born earlier and later. This, in fact, is true only as between persons born in 1917-21 who worked well beyond age 62 and those born **before** 1917 who also worked well beyond age 62.

In 1972, Congress changed the method for calculating Social Security benefits. The purpose of this change was to have inflation reflected in Social Security benefits. The 1972 law, however, did not work in the way intended because of dramatic changes in the relationship of wage and price inflation. The result was that Social Security benefits were over-indexed for inflation. Benefits soon escalated to levels much higher than Congress intended. This caused a severe strain on the financial stability of the Social Security system, and Congress soon recognized that corrective action was required.

In 1977, Congress corrected the method by which the effects of inflation are reflected in calculating Social Security benefits. The purpose was to bring benefits back to levels historically intended by Congress and avert a financial crisis for the Social Security system.

Congress faced a dilemma though on the issue of fairness. If retirement benefits were lowered only for those becoming eligible in the future, then these persons would feel unfairly disadvantaged. However, lowering benefits for those retirees already receiving benefits, or eligible to receive benefits, was considered even less fair. Congress decided to let older retirees, those born before 1917, keep their unintended windfall. People born after 1921 would have their benefits calculated under the new law.

But people born during 1917-1921, who were close to 60 when the law was passed, were given special treatment. For these so-called notch babies, the law provided two ways to calculate benefits, and beneficiaries would get whichever one was better. Benefits for the notch babies are sometime lower than for older people, because they don't get part of the accidental windfall. But benefits are sometimes better than for younger people.

Unfortunately, many of the notch babies are misinformed about the effect of the law and think they're being cheated. In fact, the opposite is true for many such recipients. The real problem: there's no good way to correct the mistake of letting benefits get too high under the 1972 law. If Congress took the windfall away from people who had already retired, it would seem unfair to people who had made financial plans based on a certain income expectation. On the other hand, if it extended the windfall to a further age group, people just under the age would complain that they deserve it too — exactly what the notch babies say.

Appealing Unfavorable Decisions

With the exception of the disability determinations, almost all Social Security claims are decided on clear-cut issues. The overwhelming majority of appeals are filed on disability claims. A claimant has 60 days from receipt of a written notice to file an appeal.

The appeal process proceeds as follows:

(1) **Reconsideration:** A reconsideration entails a complete re-examination of the claim by a different decision-maker.

(2) **Hearing:** A hearing is conducted by an administrative law judge. A claimant can appear in person at the hearing. It is at this stage that many claimants decide to be represented by an attorney.

(3) **Appeals Council Review:** Appeals Council Review involves a technical review of the decision of the administrative law judge for conformity with applicable laws and regulations.

(4) **U.S. District Court:** This is the first step of the regular federal judicial process in which a dissatisfied applicant brings suit against the government.

History of Social Security

Many factors contributed to passage of the Social Security Act of 1935. As the U.S. changed rapidly from an agricultural to an industrial economy, individuals became less self-sufficient. The Great Depression of the early 1930s caused many political leaders to believe that the time had come to enact federal legislation to relieve social problems that existed. Most other industrial nations had passed comprehensive social insurance laws many years earlier.

Payroll taxes began January 1, 1937. The rate for both employees and employers was 1% on earnings up to $3,000 per year, or a maximum tax each of $30. This tax level continued through 1949, and there were few benefit changes during this period after the very significant amendments in 1939 (see page 164). The tax increases that have taken place since then are shown on page 16; benefit increases have generally kept pace with inflation.

Congress has made amendments to Social Security many times in its long history. Some of the most significant changes follow.

1939   Benefits for dependents and survivors added to the law (page 12);

1950   Coverage extended to 10 million additional persons, primarily, nonfarm self-employed (except professionals); farm and domestic workers; U.S. citizens employed abroad by U.S. employers; federal employees not under a retirement system; employees of charitable, educational, and religious nonprofit organizations (on elective basis); and employees of state and local governments (on elective basis);

1954   Coverage extended to the farm self-employed and professionals (except doctors, dentists, and lawyers);

1956   Benefits established for disabled workers, ages 50 to 64, coverage extended to military personnel, dentists, and lawyers;

1960   Disability provisions extended to workers of all ages (pages 73-83);

1965   Medicare hospital insurance (Part A) and medical insurance (Part B) enacted (pages 101-128); coverage extended to doctors;

1972   Several types of annual automatic adjustments established. Effective each January 1, maximum taxable earnings base and the earnings limitation (retirement test) changed in accordance with pay levels. Effective each June, benefits changed, based on cost-of-living increases (page 151);

1977   Taxes increased; method of calculating benefits changed;

1980   Disability benefits for young workers and maximum family benefits in the event of disability both reduced;

1981   Minimum benefit of $122 a month eliminated; benefits for college students eliminated gradually during 1982-85;

1982   Age at which the earnings limitation no longer applies reduced from age 72 to age 70; employer-sponsored healthcare plans for employees ages 65 through 69, and their spouses, became primary payer, and Medicare the secondary payer; Medicare Part B premium established at 25% of the program cost, instead of tying changes in it to the COLA for cash benefits;

1983   Coverage extended to newly hired federal employees and on a compulsory basis to all employees of nonprofit organizations; COLA deferred for six months — to be paid each January, starting in 1984; larger increases for delayed retirement provided, beginning for persons reaching age 65 in 1990 and after (page 55); age at which full retirement benefits are paid gradually increased from 65 to 67, beginning in 2003 and reaching 67 in 2027 (page 47); retirement earnings test for persons reaching the Normal Retirement Age liberalized, beginning in 1990 (page 60); scheduled Social Security tax rate increases accelerated; up to one-half of Social Security benefits made subject to federal income taxes for persons with high income from other sources (page 24); divorced spouses permitted to draw benefits after age 62 if ex-spouse is eligible for benefits (whether or not claimed); deceased worker's earnings to be indexed (adjusted for wage inflation) for years after death in computing deferred survivor benefits;

1986   Removal of age-70 ceiling for period when employer-sponsored healthcare plan is primary to Medicare; Medicare made secondary payer for disabled employees covered by an employer-sponsored healthcare plan as a current employee, providing employer has 100 employees or more (applies to family members, as well) (page 117);

1988   Medicare Catastrophic Coverage Act enacted, expanding benefits significantly and increasing costs to beneficiaries (effective for 1989 only, because the law was repealed in late 1989);

1990   Coverage extended to state and local government employees not covered by a retirement plan of their employer; taxable earnings base for 1.45% Medicare tax increased to $125,000 for 1991 (compared to $53,400 for the 6.2% Social Security tax) (page 14); Medicare Part B deductible increased from $75 to $100; physicians limited to what they can charge Medicare patients, decreasing over three years to 115% of Medicare's allowable charges after 1992 (page 116);

1993   For 1994, and later years, taxes on Social Security benefits were increased, making up to 85% subject to federal income taxes for high-income beneficiaries; also, the earnings ceiling was removed for the 1.45% Medicare tax.

With the exception of railroad workers and some federal, state, and local government employees, virtually all workers are now covered by Social Security. Except for the fact that a portion of Medicare Part B expenses are paid from general revenues, Social Security and Medicare have not received any federal general revenues for permanent long-range features of law, but only money collected through payroll taxes, plus interest on the reserves, plus the income taxes on benefits. Such income, to the extent not needed for current benefit payments, is invested exclusively in government bonds.

The Future of Social Security

Social Security is currently quite healthy, but it faces serious long-term problems. The important 1983 amendments (see page 165), which were intended to restore financial health to the program for 75 years, have at least succeeded in the short-term. Since then, Social Security revenues have significantly outpaced expenditures. Annual payroll tax revenues are projected to continue to exceed benefit payments until 2013. From 2013 until 2030 a combination of payroll taxes, trust fund interest, and principal should enable the system to meet all of its obligations. However, under the intermediate (most likely to occur) projections in the 1995 Social Security Board of Trustees report, beginning in 2030 the system will not be able to meet all of its obligations. This is a serious problem, but it is not an immediate crisis, nor does it need to be a crisis at all. The sooner, however, that measures are taken to address these projected long-range cash-flow problems, the less drastic such measures will need to be. Adjustments that are scheduled well in advance, and implemented on a gradual or incremental basis, can make a big difference.

The projected long-term problems for Social Security are of special concern to young and middle-aged people. Many are convinced that Social Security will either not be there for them when they reach retirement age, or at best, that it will only provide a much lower level of retirement-income protection than it traditionally has.

This decline in confidence can be attributed to a number of different factors including:

- Frequent reports in the media that Social Security will eventually go bankrupt;

- The assumed unsustainability of an income-transfer program that faces a narrowing ratio of workers to beneficiaries when the generation of baby boomers retires;

- Skepticism about whether the assets held by the Social Security trust funds are of real value or are just worthless government IOUs;

- Concerns about federal budget deficits and the national debt, and how so-called "entitlement programs" contribute to these problems; and

- A widespread lack of confidence in government programs.

A number of proposals are being made to address the long-range problems of Social Security. One such proposal is to lower future COLAs. Proponents argue that the current formula overstates inflation for retirees and that small adjustments can result in tremendous long-term savings for the system. Critics argue that inflation may actually be **understated** for retirees when full consideration is given to medical expenses. They also point out that COLAs are not really benefit increases, but rather that they merely maintain the purchasing power of current benefits.

There are some groups that advocate major reforms of the current system. Some argue that the trust fund reserves should be invested in the stock market rather than in special-issue Treasury obligations. They point out that the stock market has historically provided a significantly greater real rate of return. Critics of this approach point out that a conservative investment with a predictable return devoid of large fluctuations is more suitable for a national social insurance program. They also point out that not using trust fund assets to assist in financing current government borrowing will mean that the government would have to borrow more from the private sector to make up the difference.

Another proposal receiving much attention calls for means-testing Social Security benefits. Advocates note that not only do Social Security benefits go to low- and middle-income persons, but also affluent persons receive benefits. Some characterize this as welfare for the rich. They question how we can afford to pay entitlements to the rich when we have a large national debt and a Social Security system facing insolvency. Critics of means-testing point out that Social Security is a self-funded program. Denying benefits to those persons who have paid the most into the system would be unfair and would undermine important public support for the program. Such persons already receive a smaller rate of return for their Social Security taxes than low-income persons. Excluding high-income persons would also make Social Security a welfare program and cause some stigmatization of those who receive benefits. They also point out that the means-testing of Social Security would act as a disincentive for individual savings and employer-sponsored retirement plans.

Others call for even more fundamental change. Proposals range from partial to full privatization of the system. Supporters of privatization point out that this would increase individual responsibility for retirement planning, that individuals would be able to achieve greater investment returns, and that it would cause a much needed improvement in the national savings rate. Critics argue that a privatized system would undermine the important social adequacy component of the system under which a basic floor of protection is provided for all participants through a broad pooling of risk. They also point out that proponents of privatization often overlook the important disability and survivor insurance components of the present system. Also, not everyone will be fortunate enough to realize substantial investment returns. It is also pointed out that any such major overhaul of the system would entail many transition costs which would have to be borne by the general treasury.

There are others who favor the basic approach of the present system, which balances the components of social adequacy and individual equity (generally providing greater benefits to those who have paid more into the system). They maintain that long-range solvency for the system can be achieved through moderate adjustments. They generally advocate some combination of tax increases and benefit reductions.

These traditionalists maintain that necessary increases in the payroll tax rate can be implemented in small increments and scheduled decades in advance. They further maintain that such tax increases should be far more than compensated for by the very likely greater increases in the productivity of the overall economy. They also advocate removing the special income tax treatment for Social Security benefits and taxing them the same as any other contributory pension and continuing to direct such revenues back to the Social Security trust funds. Critics argue that taxes are already too high and that any increase in taxes, even ones scheduled many years in advance, are not politically feasible.

On the benefit side of the equation, there are proposals to further gradually increase the age at which full retirement benefits are payable and/or accelerate increases already scheduled. This would not only save the system money, but it would also recognize the increasing life expectancy of retirees. There could be similar changes regarding when benefits are first payable for early retirement and the amount of the actuarial reduction for taking them early. In addition, certain technical changes in the benefit calculation formula could be implemented that would result in a slight decrease in benefit amounts. Critics argue that this will just further exacerbate the individual equity component of Social Security by increasing the length of time that it takes persons to get their money's worth from the program.

These are some of the proposals currently receiving much attention. Different groups and individuals advocate various versions and combinations of these and other proposals.

The debate on the future of Social Security is heating up. Social Security should continue to be financially strong for nearly 20 years and perhaps longer, but the long-range forecast is not so rosy. In addition to having long-range financial problems, the Social Security system must face these challenges in a political environment that increasingly doubts the effectiveness of government programs, and is reexamining the proper role of government. It is most unlikely that any major changes will be enacted before the 1996 election. However, the debate will probably intensify after that.

11

Supplemental Security Income

Supplemental Security Income (SSI), is a federal assistance program for aged (65 or older), blind, or disabled persons with little or no income and resources.

SSI is administered by the Social Security Administration; however, it is a separate program from Social Security. SSI is financed by the general revenues of the government. The Social Security trust funds are not used for SSI. The trust funds are even reimbursed from the General Treasury for the expenses which the Social Security Administration incurs for administering SSI.

The maximum federal SSI payment for an eligible individual in 1996 is $470 per month. It is $705 per month for an eligible couple. The basic SSI payment is reduced by one-third if an eligible person is living in another person's household and receiving support and maintenance in-kind from that person. The payment rate may be less if a person has other income. Many of the states supplement the federal payment. Amounts of state supplements vary. Most SSI recipients qualify for Medicaid, and many qualify for food stamps as well. Eligibility requirements for these programs can vary from state to state.

When establishing initial entitlement for SSI disability payments for adults, the same definition of disability is used as in the Social Security disability program. Disabled means that you are so severely impaired, mentally or physically, that you cannot perform any substantial gainful work. The impairment must be expected to last at least 12 months or result in earlier death. A special, broader definition of disability is used for children. There is no five month waiting period for SSI disability payments as there is for Social Security disability benefits.

Not all income and resources are counted when determining eligibility and the payment amount. Your home, car, ordinary household items, burial plot, and $1,500 face value of life insurance are generally not counted. An individual is allowed $2,000 in savings or other countable assets. A couple is allowed $3,000. There is a $20 per month income exclusion. In addition, $65 per month of **earned** income, plus one-half of the remainder of **earned** income is excluded when determining countable income. This earned income exclusion is intended to encourage those who are able to work to do so. A portion of the income and resources of ineligible spouses and parents who live in the same household is considered when determining the countable income of an SSI applicant or recipient.

An aged, blind, or disabled person who receives a small Social Security benefit may also qualify for SSI.

Example: Ms. Adams is 65 and receives a gross Social Security benefit (before deduction for the Medicare B premium) of $370. She has no other income and meets all other requirements for SSI eligibility. She can receive $120 in SSI payments.

$370.00	Social Security benefit (gross)
− 20.00	Income exclusion
$350.00	Countable income
$470.00	Maximum SSI payment rate
− 350.00	Countable income
$120.00	SSI payment

In this example, her gross monthly income is $490 ($370.00 Social Security and $120.00 SSI). Her net monthly income is $447.50 after she has her Part B premium of $42.50 deducted from her Social Security benefit.

In addition, Ms. Adams should contact her state or local medical assistance office to see if she qualifies for Medicaid, or if she is eligible to be a Qualified Medicare Beneficiary so that the state will pay her Part B monthly premium for her. If she qualifies, then her net monthly income will increase by $42.50 for a total of $490.

If you know someone who might qualify for SSI, you should encourage them to contact the Social Security Administration right away and apply for benefits. There is no provision to pay any retroactive SSI before the effective filing date.

SSI payments are normally issued on the first day of the month, representing payment for that month. If the first is on a Saturday, Sunday, or holiday, then payment is made on the preceding business day.

12

Things To Do

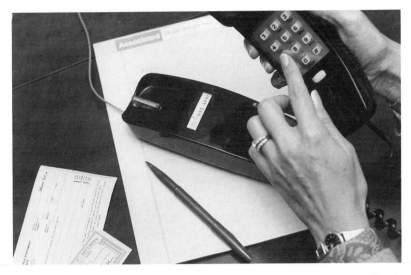

You should do several things to make sure you get all the benefits to which you are entitled. Some of these things should be done now. Others should be done later.

Remember this: Social Security will not start your benefits until you file an application. Start with a telephone call to the Social Security Administration's national toll-free number: **800-772-1213.** Most applications can be taken by phone.

If you are late in filing an application, you may not be paid all of the benefits which you could have received.

When To Do It	What To Do

Now

- Everyone (even children) should have a Social Security number and a card showing that number. It's needed when you buy a government bond, open a savings account, and especially when you get a job. The law requires a child, regardless of age, to have a Social Security a number in order to be claimed as a dependent on an income tax return. If you have a number but have lost the card, apply for a new card but not a new number. If you have forgotten your number, the Social Security Administration can find it. Call them.

- Complete and mail Form SSA-7004 attached in this book. The form is labeled "Request for Earnings and Benefit Estimate Statement." Sign the form before mailing it.

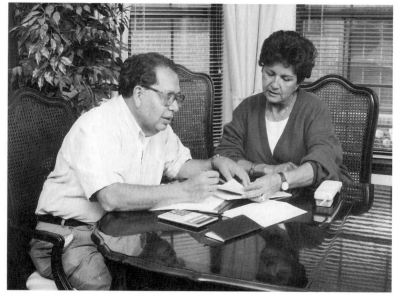

When you receive your Earnings and Benefit Estimate Statement

- As soon as you receive the Statement, check the earnings information for errors. If you find an error, call Social Security.

When you file your federal income tax return

- If you have had more than one job and earned more than the maximum for Social Security for that year, you probably paid excess taxes. You should claim a credit for these excess taxes when you file your federal income tax return. Your W-2 forms show how much you paid. Look at the boxes labeled "Social Security tax withheld."

Periodically

- You should request your Earnings and Benefit Estimate Statement once every three years. This is especially important if you have changed employers, or if you have more than one employer. Social Security may have difficulty correcting errors that occurred long ago. If you identify an error early, you will usually be able to get it corrected easily.

Before you file for benefits

- Because you do not know when disability or death claims might have to be filed, why not get papers ready now? Make sure you have a certified copy of your birth certificate. Social Security cannot use ordinary photocopies. If you are filing for benefits based on your spouse's or former spouse's PIA, you may need to present a certified copy of your marriage certificate. If you apply for benefits as a divorced spouse, you will also need your divorce decree.

Three months or more before you start benefits

- File an application. Processing an application takes time. Always start the process at least three months before the date you want retirement benefits to begin. To be safe, do so in the January before you intend to retire, but not earlier than four months before you turn 62. Disability or survivor benefits should be filed for as soon as possible after disability or death occurs. Any application can be started by calling the Social Security Administration's national toll free number 800-772-1213.

If you think a decision by Social Security is wrong

- If you believe that a decision by Social Security is wrong, you can appeal within 60 days. Start by calling Social Security. They will tell you how to have your case reviewed. Several levels of appeal are possible within the Social Security Administration. After that, you can appeal to the federal courts, but you will need a lawyer.

Any time

- If you think you may be eligible for benefits, file an application. **Don't just ask** if you are eligible. An informal question is never given the attention that an application receives. If an application is incorrectly denied, its filing date will be used when your benefits do start.

After you retire

- After you start receiving benefits, if your earnings exceed the Earnings Limitation (pages 60-64), call Social Security and report this information to them. Having benefits withheld is less painful than having to pay back benefits that should not have been paid to you. And if benefits are paid incorrectly, you **will** have to pay them back. In addition, the law provides penalties for intentionally failing to report your earnings or reporting them incorrectly.

When you reach age 70

- The Earnings Limitation does not apply beginning with the month you reach age 70. You can then earn any amount without losing any benefits.

If disabled

- File your application promptly so that it can be processed during the waiting period. Cooperate with any instructions regarding rehabilitation services. If you have a good reason not to do what is requested, call Social Security and discuss it with them. All earnings from work must be reported if you are receiving disability benefits.

Mother or father

- If you are receiving benefits because you have a child in your care, and the child leaves your care, report it at once. Payments made improperly **will** have to be repaid.

If you lose your card

- Call Social Security and give them all the information they request. They will arrange for you to receive a new card with the same number. **Do not apply for a new number.** A record of all your earnings is filed under this number. You should be sure that you receive credit for all your work.

**When you
are close to
retirement age**

- If you can choose the time to retire, look carefully at the Earnings Limitation. You may be able to start your benefits effective January 1 and keep on working until you have earned the annual Earnings Limitation (page 60) before actually stopping work. In this case, you would lose no benefits at all.

**If you travel
outside the U.S.**

- Remember that Medicare does not usually pay for hospital or other medical expenses outside the U.S. (exceptions are Canadian and Mexican facilities if they are nearest to your home or while traveling to or from Alaska through Canada). If you plan to travel abroad, investigate other insurance.

**If you become
eligible for a
second benefit**

- Sometimes you can become eligible for a benefit on someone else's work record even though you are already receiving a benefit on your own record. Call Social Security and tell them all the facts. Tell them you want to file an application. When they know about both benefits, they will figure both, and you will get the larger one. If they do not know about one benefit because you do not apply, they cannot check to see if you should be receiving more.

Remember
- Social Security will not ordinarily look for you to pay you a benefit. They will not take any action until you apply. Then they will process your application carefully and with reasonable speed, considering that over 43 million people now receive Social Security benefits each month.

You have to apply for your benefit.

13

Frequently Asked Questions — and the Answers!

Q. Will I receive Social Security benefits on my own Social Security work record or on my spouse's? Can I get both?

A. If you are eligible for more than one type of benefit at the same time, the most you can receive is the equivalent of the higher benefit. When you apply for benefits, Social Security will automatically calculate all possible benefits for which you are eligible. If you are eligible for both a retirement benefit and a spouse's benefit, then you will receive the retirement benefit and the excess, if any, by which the spouse's benefit exceeds the retirement benefit. If you are eligible for both a retirement benefit and a surviving spouse's benefit, then again the most you can receive is the equivalent of the higher benefit. In this situation, however, you can receive a reduced benefit on one Social Security record and then switch to an unreduced benefit, if higher, on the other Social Security record at or near your Normal Retirement Age (currently 65). Social Security will calculate all possible options and advise you accordingly.

Q. If I retire before I am old enough for Social Security, what effect will this have on the amount of my future Social Security benefit?

A. People who work continually from their early twenties and retire in their mid to late fifties will find that early retirement has only a minimal effect on the average earnings used to compute their Social Security benefit. Social Security retirement benefits are determined by career average earnings subject to the Social Security tax.

The 35 highest years of earnings are considered for people born after 1928. If you work fewer than 35 years, then some years of zero earnings will be averaged in. If you work more than 35 years, then the low years of earnings in excess of 35 will be dropped from consideration. Earnings in years prior to age 60 are indexed to reflect wage inflation. Actual earnings are used after age 59.

Q.   I have earned the maximum required 40 credits. Does this mean that I get the maximum Social Security retirement benefit?

A.   No. Having 40 credits means that you are insured for a Social Security retirement benefit. The amount of your benefit is determined by your career average earnings covered by Social Security, and the age at which you begin receiving benefits.

Q.   My ex-husband and I were divorced several years ago after more than 10 years of marriage. We are both age 62. He worked in a much higher paying job than I did. Can I receive Social Security divorced spouse's benefits on his work record?

A.   Yes, assuming that you are not currently remarried, and that you are not entitled to a higher benefit on any other Social Security work record, including your own. It does not matter if he is remarried. Nor does he have to have started receiving his own benefits yet, as long as he is eligible for benefits. If you were still married, you could not start spouse's benefits on his work record until he started his own.

Q. I am the ex-husband in the previous question. I am remarried. Does the Social Security spouse benefit paid to my ex-wife in any way reduce the amount of benefits payable to me or my current wife?

A. No.

Q. I do not have enough credits to qualify for Social Security benefits. Can I voluntarily pay Social Security taxes to earn additional credits?

A. No. You can only earn Social Security credits by working in covered employment or self-employment. This is consistent with the overall purpose of the program, which is to help replace the earnings which are lost due to retirement, disability, or death.

Q. If I start collecting Social Security retirement benefits when I turn 62, when do I get my first check?

A. Entitlement to retirement or aged spouse benefits cannot begin until the first full month that you are age 62. If your birthday is on the first or second day of the month, then you are considered to be 62 throughout the month of your birthday. If your birthday is after the second of the month, then the following month is the first full month that you are 62. Your first check is not normally due until the third day of the month following your month of entitlement. If the third of the month is on a Saturday, Sunday, or holiday, then the check is due on the preceding business day.

Example 1: 62nd birthday on April 1 or 2. Your first month of entitlement is April and your first benefit check is normally due on May 3.

Example 2: 62nd birthday on April 3. Your first month of entitlement is May and your first benefit check is normally due on June 3.

Q. My father died on the last day of January. Can we keep the Social Security benefit that arrived for him on February 3?

A. No. The check received on February 3 is actually the benefit for January. Benefits are not due for the month of death. If he had died on February 1, then he would have lived throughout the month of January and the benefit check could be reissued to an eligible survivor, or if none, then to the estate.

Q. I am 62, retired, financially well off, and don't need Social Security retirement benefits to meet my current expenses. Should I go ahead and elect to receive reduced benefits beginning at age 62 or should I wait until I'm 65 and receive the full benefit amount?

A. There is no simple answer to this question. Retirees have to make their own informed decisions. Retirement benefits are permanently reduced $\frac{5}{9}$ of 1% for each month of entitlement to benefits prior to age 65. This currently equals a 20% reduction at age 62. (See page 47 for scheduled increases in the normal retirement age for people born after 1937.) Persons who choose to start their benefits before age 65 receive less per month than they would receive by waiting until 65, but they will of course, receive benefits for a longer period of time. The initial advantage of receiving reduced benefits will keep a person ahead, in terms of total lifetime benefits received, for 15 years. The initial advantage lasts until age 77 for a person who starts benefits at age 62, and it lasts until age 80 for a person who starts benefits at age 64 years and 11 months. If the unneeded benefits are saved or invested, then any accumulated interest or investment gain will increase the initial advantage. If income taxes are due on benefits received, then this will also have an effect.

And finally, one's health condition and the resulting life expectancy will be a major factor of consideration. The current life expectancy for a person who is 65 is about 15 years for a man and 18½ years for a woman. (See pages 52-55 for a detailed discussion.)

Q. Is the money in the Social Security trust funds used for other government programs besides Social Security?

A. Indirectly, yes.

By law, the revenues from Social Security taxes can only be used to pay for Social Security benefits and the administrative expenses of the program, which average only about 1% of benefits. Any excess must be invested in U.S. government securities. Both the principal and interest on these securities is guaranteed by the full faith and credit of the United States. When the Social Security trust funds buy these U.S. government securities, they are loaning the money to the government and thus helping to finance the national debt in the same manner as anyone else who buys a treasury bill or savings bond. The government in turn uses this borrowed money to pay the costs for many other government programs.

This is similar in principle to the situation of a person who deposits money into a savings account. The financial institution agrees to repay the principal plus interest to the depositor. The financial institution takes that money and lends it to someone else, who may use that money to buy a home or a car. In that sense, the person who deposited money into a savings account is indirectly financing someone else's purchase of a home or car.

Q.   I was seriously injured in an accident and I am now disabled and unable to return to work. I have heard that there is a five or six month waiting period for Social Security disability. I have also heard that you have to be disabled a year to qualify for disability. This is all very confusing. When should I apply to the Social Security Administration for disability benefits?

A.   You should apply now!

One of the requirements to qualify for disability benefits is that the disability must be expected to last at least 12 months or result in earlier death. This doesn't mean that the disability has actually lasted for 12 months, but rather that it is expected to last at least 12 months.

There is a waiting period of five full calendar months after the onset of disability before entitlement to benefits can begin. In effect, this often means six months or in some cases almost seven months. For example, if you became disabled on January 2, then the five full months of your waiting period would be February through June. In this example, July would be the first month of entitlement and the benefit check for July would not normally be due until August 3.

Also, the disability claim process can be very lengthy. It usually takes the Social Security Administration at least three months to process a disability claim. Furthermore, a large percentage of claims are only approved upon appeal after having originally been denied. Thus, it is very important to apply as soon as possible.

Q. I am age 66 and receive Social Security surviving spouse benefits. If I remarry, will I lose my benefits?

A. No. Remarriage does not terminate surviving spouse benefits to widows or widowers age 60 and older, or disabled widows and widowers age 50 and older. Remarriage before attaining the minimum age to qualify for benefits does preclude entitlement to surviving spouse benefits as long as the subsequent marriage continues. If the subsequent marriage should end in death or divorce, then entitlement to benefits on the prior spouse's work record is permitted. (See pages 154-155 for a detailed discussion.)

Young widows and widowers who are entitled to benefits because they care for a child lose their benefits if they remarry. However, the child's benefits are unaffected by the remarriage of the parent.

Q. Why does the Social Security annual earnings test penalize the person who works, but not the person who has substantial investment income? This seems very unfair.

A. Unlike welfare, Social Security is not a means tested program. Social Security retirement benefits are intended to be insurance for loss of income due to retirement, not as insurance for attaining age 65.

Social Security is not designed to be a person's only source of retirement income. Rather, it is intended to provide a base of income to which the retired person can add other sources of retirement income such as private pensions, savings, and other investments. By not considering investment income for purposes of the earnings test, individual savings is encouraged.

Q. My wife and I will visit Europe this summer. Will Medicare cover us over there if we require emergency medical treatment?

A. No. Medicare does not cover medical treatment received outside of the United States except in certain cases of emergency treatment along the U.S. borders with Canada and Mexico or in Canada while traveling between Alaska and the "lower 48" states. If you have other health insurance, you should check to see if that policy provides foreign travel protection.

Q. Are Medicare and Medicaid the same thing?

A. No.

Medicare is a federal program of health insurance for eligible people age 65 and older, Social Security disability beneficiaries who have been entitled to monthly benefits for two years, and eligible persons with kidney failure. Financial status is not a factor of eligibility. You apply with the Social Security Administration for entitlement to Medicare.

Medicaid is a joint federal/state program of medical assistance for eligible people with low income and resources. Applications for Medicaid are filed with the state or local Medicaid office or public assistance office.

Q. I will soon be 65. I am already retired, and I receive Social Security benefits. I have very good health insurance protection from my former employer. Do I need to enroll in Part B of Medicare and pay the monthly premium?

A. Generally yes, but not always. If the only employer sponsored health insurance you have is from the employer that you have retired from, then yes, you generally do need Part B. Your retiree health insurance will ordinarily revert to a Medicare supplement when you attain age 65.

However, if your spouse still works for an employer with 20 or more employees, and you have health insurance coverage under your spouse's employer sponsored health insurance plan, then the law requires that plan to remain as your primary health insurance. In this situation, you probably would not need to enroll in Part B until your spouse retires. You would, however, want to determine if there are any gaps in that coverage which Part B could fill and whether the additional benefit coverage is worth the Part B premium cost.

Q. My wife and I both receive Social Security benefits. My benefit is higher. If I die first, how much will her widow's benefit be?

A. If she is at least 65 when you die, then her total benefit will be what your benefit was, or in some cases slightly higher. It can be less if she is younger than 65 when you die.

Q. I retired last year at age 68 and started receiving my Social Security benefits. My wife, who is not insured for benefits on her own work record, became entitled to a spouse's benefit on my work record when she was 66. Why is her benefit less than one-half of mine? Both of us waited until after age 65 to start our Social Security. I thought her benefit was supposed to be one-half of mine.

A. Your benefit is increased because you earned Delayed Retirement Credits. You earned a DRC for each month that you did not receive a benefit after attaining age 65. These DRC's are applied only to your benefit, not to your wife's. If you die first, however, these DRC's will be used to increase the amount of the survivor benefit payable to your wife. (See page 55 for the various DRC rates based on different years of birth.)

Q. My parents are over 65 and have never lived in the U.S. They are considering moving to the U.S. to be closer to me. Even though they are not eligible for monthly Social Security benefits, can they enroll in Medicare?

A. No, at least not right away. They will, however, be eligible to enroll in Medicare on a premium-payment basis either if they become U.S. citizens, or if they are lawfully admitted for permanent residence and have resided in the U.S. continuously for five years. They can enroll either for Parts A and B, or for Part B only. They cannot just take Part A.

The monthly premium rates in 1996 are $289 for Part A and $42.50 for Part B. These monthly premium rates will increase in future years.

Q. My wife and I have both worked in high-paying jobs. We will each be eligible for Social Security retirement benefits based on our own work records. Will our combined benefits be limited by a family maximum?

A. No. The family maximum rule can only apply when multiple benefits are payable on the same Social Security work record.

Q. What is SSI?

A. SSI stands for Supplemental Security Income. SSI is a federal program of financial assistance to the aged (age 65 or older), blind, and disabled who have little or no income and resources. Even though SSI is administered by the Social Security Administration, it is a different program than Social Security, and it is funded from general revenues, not from Social Security taxes (pages 172-174).

William M. Mercer, Incorporated, is the world's largest compensation and employee-benefits consulting firm. We have offices in 43 U.S. cities. Worldwide, the Mercer organization has about 7,400 employees and offices in 107 cities in 26 countries. As we have expanded geographically, we have also increased services to meet clients' needs.

Other Social Security and Medicare information services include:

- 48-page Social Security booklet;
- 32-page Social Security booklet;
- Medicare booklet;
- quarterly newsletter;
- consulting services;
- training seminars;
- audio-visual programs;
- "giveaway" brochures and booklets for life insurance companies and training programs for agents.

Index

195